Out-of-Hospital Transfusion Therapy

Out-of-Hospital Transfusion Therapy

Editors

Joy L. Fridey, MD
Associate Medical Director
Blood Bank of San Bernardino
and Riverside Counties
San Bernardino, California

Christina A. Kasprisin, MS, RN
Lecturer
College of Nursing
University of Vermont
South Burlington, Vermont

Linda A. Issitt, MT(ASCP)SBB
Pheresis Coordinator
Pediatric Bone Marrow Transplant Program
Duke University Medical Center
Durham, North Carolina

American Association of Blood Banks
Bethesda, Maryland
1994

American Association of Blood Banks
8101 Glenbrook Road
Bethesda, Maryland 20814-2749

ISBN NO. 1-56395-029-4
Printed in the United States

Text paper meets EPA guidelines for minimum recovered material content (50% recycled fiber, including 10% postconsumer waste)

Technical/Scientific Workshops Committee

Ronald A. Sacher, MD, Chairman

James P. AuBuchon, MD
Frederick B. Axelrod, MD
Mark E. Brecher, MD
Daniel B. Brubaker, DO
Linda A. Chambers, MD
Joy L. Fridey, MD
Linda A. Issitt, MT(ASCP)SBB
Leigh C. Jefferies, MD
Susan T. Johnson, MT(ASCP)SBB
Sanford R. Kurtz, MD
Barbara Laird-Fryer, MT(ASCP)SBB
Douglas M. Smith, MD, PhD
Steven D. Sosler, MS, SBB(ASCP)
Sally G. Swenson-Caglioti, MT(ASCP)SBB
Susan M. Wilson, MT(ASCP)SBB
Laura Lee Woods, MS, MT(ASCP)SBB

Contents

Foreword

The last 15 years have brought about a dramatic revolution in health-care delivery and reimbursement. The paradigm of complicated care being rendered almost exclusively in inpatient settings has inexorably begun to shift. Driven predominantly by cost and, to a lesser degree, customer service considerations, many procedures and treatments that were considered to be the domain of tertiary-care centers are now being performed with increasing frequency in short-stay and outpatient units, urgent care centers, physicians' offices and patients' homes. Added to now-routine types of home care treatments such as hyperalimentation and chemotherapy is transfusion therapy. Home transfusion has been able to evolve, in part, because in an effort to expand their services and respond to the need for more home-based care, a few blood centers and hospital blood banks began years ago to function as transfusion services by providing blood for home transfusion through home health agencies.

In 1985 the AABB published its first monograph on out-of-hospital transfusion. Since that time, a growing number of blood centers and hospital blood banks have developed out-of-hospital transfusion programs. What was an emerging trend in the 1980s has become a sought-after clinical service in the 1990s. Organizations aspiring to provide these services and those already participating are asking for guidance on issues ranging from the logistics of setting up a program to regulation. In response to these solicitations, the AABB is offering this new monograph on out-of-hospital transfusion therapy.

The six chapters in this text encompass those areas that are deemed key to addressing the many issues that organizations must consider when deciding to enter this patient care arena. It is assumed that the readership will predominantly be composed of blood bankers, and most of the content and manner of presentation reflect this. However, the intended audience also includes organizations that have not traditionally provided transfusion services, and the chapters take into account their educational needs as well.

The chapters covering the perspectives of blood centers, hospital transfusion services and home health agencies get down to the logistical "nitty gritty" and could serve as useful resources for institutions setting up or running an out-of-hospital transfusion service. It is important that legal and financial issues be considered when establishing a program, and both of these areas merit special consideration in the form of separate chapters.

Finally, because there is a growing chorus of voices calling for regulatory guidance, a chapter on regulation has been included. It is appropriate to note here that with the exception of one state, there currently are no comprehensive federal, state or other regulations that apply to all aspects of out-of-hospital transfusion. The inclusion of a chapter on regulation is not to be interpreted as endorsement of or a call for regulation, but is intended to prompt readers to look closely at their own programs and determine if good transfusion practice is being followed. It is the philosophy of the text editors and many in the blood banking profession that if blood providers and transfusionists adhere to already-established standards of transfusion practice, the imposition of regulations by external agencies will not be necessary.

It is the hope of those contributing that this text will serve as a welcome and indispensable reference to institutions participating in the provision of out-of-hospital transfusion services.

Joy L. Fridey, MD
Christina A. Kasprisin, MS, RN
Linda A. Issitt, MT(ASCP)SBB
Editors

In: Fridey JL, Kasprisin CA and Issitt LA, eds.
Out-of-Hospital Transfusion Therapy
Bethesda, MD: American Association of Blood Banks, 1994

1

Medical Aspects of Home Blood Transfusion: A View from the Hospital

Edward L. Snyder, MD

A HOME BLOOD TRANSFUSION program is intended to provide patients with traditional hemotherapy services in an out-of-hospital setting.[1-5] Establishing such a program is an appropriate consideration in today's reorganizing health-care system where outpatient and out-of-hospital therapies are replacing inpatient procedures. Transfusion of a patient in a nonhospital setting (at home), however, is fraught with medicolegal concerns. This chapter addresses some of these issues and describes how a home transfusion program provided by a hospital can be designed to be safe and effective for the patient and the hospital alike. Each program that is established will need to deal with most of the issues discussed. However, some local concerns are not covered in this chapter. In such cases, the responsible medical director should assume as a guideline that, whatever the issue, the highest standards of safe transfusion practice should be followed. This principle must never be modified for the sake of convenience, collegiality or financial considerations.

Starting a Program

For a hospital that decides to offer a home transfusion program, several options are available:

Edward L. Snyder, MD, Professor of Laboratory Medicine, Yale University School of Medicine and Director, Blood Bank, Yale-New Haven Hospital, New Haven, Connecticut

1. The hospital can act solely as a blood bank and supply the needed red cells, plasma or platelets directly to private physicians, who can then arrange to have the components infused.
2. The hospital can supply blood to outside nursing agencies, which will arrange for the transfusion.
3. The hospital can run the entire program and not only supply the blood product, but also provide the nursing staff and all related aspects of the infusion process.

Regardless of how a hospital chooses to participate in a home transfusion program, it cannot abrogate the responsibilities that are inherent in its decision to supply blood, namely, to ensure that the blood transfusion is indicated, that it is administered properly and that safe transfusion practices are being followed. Thus, a hospital that supplies blood for home transfusion must have input into the medical, nursing and regulatory issues related to the transfusion program. The major initial concern is the indication for transfusion.

Obtaining Initial Approval for Home Transfusion

All requests for home blood transfusion when components are supplied by a hospital should be approved by a hospital-based physician, most appropriately the blood bank medical director, who should function as a gatekeeper. The blood bank director should ensure that the indications for transfusion are reasonable, that the appropriate medical requirements are fulfilled, and that the patient is not being placed at undue risk by receiving the transfusion at home.[6-9] This oversight role will decrease the possibility that patients are transfused at home for what could be considered questionable reasons. Where appropriate, the chairperson of the hospital transfusion committee could also function in this capacity.

This author's institution supplies blood for home transfusion only for physicians who are on its own medical staff. This decreases the likelihood of system abuses that might occur with physicians who are not known to the hospital, and who may not be well-versed in appropriate transfusion practice. By restricting home transfusion program access to its own staff, the hospital decreases abuse in the system and also maintains greater control over who is transfusing blood from its blood bank. The hospital supplies blood only to an approved Visiting Nurses' Association (VNA) or to an acceptable home health-care agency.[10] These agencies must have their nursing staff trained in blood administration by the hospital blood bank staff and their standard operating procedures (SOPs) approved and accepted by the hospital blood bank and transfusion committee.

Identifying Suitable Patients

Home transfusion patients will have diagnoses as varied as the spectrum of medical disease. The typical home transfusion patient is an oncology patient who is anemic or thrombocytopenic, not acutely ill, and for whom transportation to the hospital would pose a significant hardship.[11] Anemic or thrombocytopenic patients who have AIDS, end-stage malignancy, or extensive inflammatory, collagen-vascular or other debilitating diseases (including neuromuscular disorders) may also be suitable candidates. Nonambulatory patients who would require a car or an ambulance to take them back and forth to the hospital fall in the acceptable category. Individuals who, only for reasons of mere convenience, prefer to be transfused at home are *not* suitable candidates for the program. Patients with hemoglobinopathies, such as sickle cell anemia or thalassemia, may also be suitable candidates. Regardless of the precautions taken, home transfusion places the recipient at greater risk than does transfusion in an inpatient or outpatient ambulatory setting. It is the philosophy of this author's institution and some other transfusion medicine specialists that if at all possible, only patients who were previously transfused without incident in a hospital setting should be considered as candidates for home transfusion. Home transfusion patients should have a stable cardiorespiratory status. They should not show signs of acute congestive heart failure or other cardiopulmonary diseases that would make transfusion at home much more dangerous.

Children can be cared for in a home transfusion program as well. In fact, because home transfusion provokes less anxiety, many children may prefer being transfused at home. The same rules proscribing home transfusion for adults for reasons of mere convenience, however, must also be applied to pediatric patients.

Individuals with hemophilia A and B have been infusing Factor VIII or Factor IX in home therapy programs for years. While these plasma derivative programs are considered safe, red cell transfusions pose a greater hazard because the red cell is a particulate antigen, and the risk of a fatal hemolytic transfusion reaction is ever-present. With particulate antigens such as red cells, transfusion of incompatible blood could produce complement fixation with resulting hemoglobinemia, hemoglobinuria, bronchospasm, shock and tubular necrosis leading to acute renal failure.[7,12] This risk is not associated with transfusion of soluble plasma antigens in products such as fresh frozen plasma, cryoprecipitate or coagulation factor concentrates.

A major safety concern regarding home transfusion lies in the accuracy and reliability of the crossmatch. Crossmatching requires mixing the patient's serum and donor red cells in a test tube in an attempt to mimic, in vitro, the in-vivo response to a transfusion. An incompatible crossmatch implies that the blood will not survive in vivo and may cause an untoward reaction. A lack of in-vitro reactivity, either agglutination or hemolysis, implies that the transfused red cells will likely survive in vivo and the transfusion will be uneventful. Although this latter assumption is almost always accurate, the risk exists that some potential serologic posttransfusion incompatibility may not be observed in vitro because the antibody titer is too low to be detected and/or the serologic techniques used are too insensitive.

Blood found to be incompatible should not be transfused in a home setting. Although this may seem obvious, many patients take medications or have immunologic disorders associated with panagglutinins. Patients with a history of multiple prior transfusions or pregnancies may have weakly reactive leukoagglutinins, presumably directed against HLA or other white cell antigens. Such a patient's crossmatches may all be weakly incompatible. Because this incompatibility may also be due to unidentified alloantibodies, it is most prudent to avoid transfusing blood to patients in a home setting if any degree of serologic incompatibility exists. If such blood "must" be transfused in the home, it should be filtered through a leukocyte reduction filter and, as some transfusion experts prefer, washed before transfusion to decrease the confusion that might be caused by a febrile or allergic transfusion reaction. The final decision to transfuse, and what to transfuse, however, is also the responsibility of the blood bank medical director or the physician responsible for administering the home transfusion program; the decision should not rest solely with the patient's private physician.

To decrease risks associated with a home transfusion program, patients transfused at home should not have a history of transfusion reactions such as recurrent fever and chills, allergic reactions or anaphylactic reactions. Problems such as pain at the IV site, lightheadedness or nausea are seen in hospitalized patients during blood infusion. Although such reactions might be considered minor in a hospital setting, a patient experiencing such reactions in a home environment could present a diagnostic dilemma for the attending nurse. This may result not only in unnecessary termination of the transfusion but also in emergency transfer of the patient to the hospital. To avoid these minor reactions as well as more classic febrile or allergic reactions, it is recommended that all units of red cells transfused at home be leukocyte-reduced or washed. Although the cost:benefit ratio of this approach must be evaluated for each individual program, the potential for incurring substantial added expenses if a febrile reaction needs to be evaluated in the hospital favors use of some form of leukocyte removal.

Leukocyte-reduction or microaggregate removal filters used to remove white cells may decrease the incidence of febrile reactions; however, their use will not remove plasma proteins that can cause allergic reactions. Washing of the red cells, however, will remove most plasma proteins. The home transfusion program medical director should consider each patient's transfusion history and current medical problems in deciding whether home transfusion is in the best interest of that patient. Patients who have clinically severe febrile or allergic transfusion reactions despite the use of leukocyte-reduced/washed blood should not be transfused in a home setting.[13-18]

Administrative Concerns

Approval of the home transfusion request by the blood bank medical director decreases the chance of inappropriate use of this service. When the author's facility receives a request from an agency to provide home blood transfusion services, hospital personnel meet with agency representatives and review their SOPs to ensure that they meet the hospital's criteria. The nurses who are part of the transfusion agency and who will administer the blood must pass the hospital transfusion training program, which includes several hours of didactic lectures, and evaluation and observation of their transfusion practices in the hospital outpatient transfusion unit. This results in the nurses being "certified" by the blood bank for a finite period of time—currently five years—showing that they have passed the hospital transfusion course. The benefits of this approach are more highly trained nurses and, if some untoward transfusion event occurs during an infusion, the ability of the hospital to document appropriate training for the nurses administering the blood in the transfusion program.

Patient identification systems must be in place. Wristbands must be provided; either hand-written or commercially furnished identification bands can be used. Some mechanism for obtaining emergency help must be available such as the ability to request assistance by calling "911" or arrangements with a local ambulance company. This will ensure that the nursing personnel will have appropriate medical back-up. The hospital requires that English-speaking relatives or friends be in the house to assist the nurse if there is a problem. This is not the primary responsibility of the hospital, but someone must be designated to ensure that these issues have been addressed and show that a system is in place. There should be limits set on the number and volume of components that can be administered at any one time, how the blood is stored and whether to use electromechanical transfusion devices, such as pumps or warmers. There must be some mechanism for hospital review of the patients' charts after transfusion. While the blood bank director approves the transfusions, the transfusion committee is the oversight committee. This administrative approach provides a forum, if needed, for discussion among the physician who wishes to provide home transfusion services and the blood bank, the nursing agency and the hospital. It spreads the responsibility for quality assurance among several individuals, and ensures that the blood bank has more "clout" when dealing with uncooperative physicians or nursing agencies. The transfusion committee is also responsible for oversight of any transfusion reactions that occur. Because transfusion committees meet on a quarterly basis at the author's institution, the blood bank director acts as its interim representative to review these issues. If there are any untoward concerns, an emergency meeting of the transfusion committee could be convened.

One must never assume that a home transfusion program will involve no risk. However, it can be made as low risk as possible by attention to detail and by appropriate review of each aspect of the program. Regardless of the hospital's best motives or intentions, legal liability is something that should be evaluated thoroughly by the risk management sections of hospitals wishing to supply blood, to ensure compliance with local and state laws.

Competition Issues

Should hospitals compete for patients in this arena or should they try to discourage home transfusion in favor of outpatient transfusion in hospital clinics? Outpatient transfusion in hospital-based clinics is preferred by many because it is safer to transfuse blood in an outpatient clinic than in the home, despite the amount of blood that is reported to be safely transfused in the home.[3,4,5,10,11] If there are medical personnel onsite, it is generally considered safer than if there is just one nurse, in a home, at a distance from the hospital. The author's hospital provides blood for outside home transfusion nursing agencies as well as for its own outpatient clinical needs. The nature of modern competitive, patient-oriented medical care ensures that sooner or later home transfusion will be requested to fill a perceived health-care need.

Program Rationale

Why should a hospital provide home transfusion services? There are several reasons, most of them economic.

1. It provides a service to the physicians on the staff at the hospital. This increases physician loyalty and strengthens ties to physicians who may have the option of transferring or admitting patients to different hospitals in a given local area.
2. It provides increased convenience (care) to patients so that these patients (customers/clients) will not want or need to go elsewhere to get desired medical services.
3. It is possible, because a home transfusion service is an outpatient program, that it might generate an excess of revenue over expenses, which may be attractive to some institutions. However, one must always remain cognizant that an improperly operated home transfusion service is an extreme liability. Failure to provide appropriate quality assurance and control can result in legal liability, which could be financially counterproductive.

Office Transfusion

Other types of outpatient transfusion settings include office transfusion or transfusion in a free-standing medical clinic. Office transfusions can be viewed as a variant of home transfusion. That is, hospitals are requested to provide blood for physicians for transfusion, in their offices. This may be appropriate because this service is most often requested by hematologists or oncologists. Any hospital providing blood for off-site physician offices, however, must remain vigilant and mindful of the fact that the mere presence of a physician in the office does not mean that the hospital can in any way be less concerned than it would be with providing blood for a nursing agency. Accordingly, the doctors and their nurses should be evaluated for suitability and competency for providing office-based transfusions. In addition to being on the hospital medical staff, the credentials and transfusion practices of the physician and his/her office should be evaluated to ensure that they are following good medical practices. The quantity and the nature of the transfusions should be reviewed by the blood bank director, to ensure that they are following safe transfusion practice. It should be ensured that any long-term storage occurs only in a *monitored* blood bank refrigerator and any short-term storage is only in an insulated portable carrier such as described below. Adhesive ("stick-on") temperature devices are available for monitoring out-of-refrigerator temperatures. Waste disposal issues apply to office-based transfusions as well as home-based transfusions.

Free-Standing Clinics

In some free-standing clinics, or surgicenters, complicated surgeries are frequently performed. Thus, doctors may wish to have blood available so that they may perform more extensive procedures such as liposuction on an outpatient basis. Such practices raise even greater concerns because blood may need to be stored without being used. To some degree, this may force the hospital supplying blood to assume greater liability. If a surgicenter wishes to store blood, it must do so in a monitored blood bank refrigerator, and there may be local, state and federal regulations that govern this practice. It is critical that a hospital blood transfusion service not distribute blood to any institution—be it a physician's office, free-standing medical clinic or home health-care agency—without having detailed knowledge of the requesting agency's SOPs. It probably would be prudent for a blood bank physician or other health-care professional to travel periodically to the doctor's office or clinic to observe a transfusion being performed and to consider on-site inspections of the doctor's office or the free-standing clinic, much the same way that the AABB inspects hospital transfusion services. Waste disposal issues as described below apply here, too.

Indications for Components

Component therapy has become the standard by which patients are transfused. Only the specific part of blood required is given, thus avoiding transfusion of unneeded blood elements. Depending on the individual's needs, one or more components may be indicated. The following paragraphs describe component composition and indications for their use in the home transfusion setting.

Whole Blood

The primary indication for whole blood transfusion is for treatment of actively bleeding patients who are likely to, or are currently suffering from, hemorrhagic shock. Usually, these patients have lost more than 25% of their total blood volume. Accordingly, use of whole blood in a home transfusion therapy program is usually inappropriate, because patients *requiring* whole blood need urgent and intensive medical care, available only in the hospital. Transfusion of whole blood to anemic patients with a normal blood volume may precipitate acute hypervolemia and pulmonary edema.

Red Blood Cells/Additive Solution Red Blood Cells

Red Blood Cells/Additive Solution Red Blood Cell units (RBCs/AS-RBCs) are indicated for chronically anemic patients who have a decreased red cell mass but who are normovolemic. RBCs are prepared from units of Whole Blood by centrifugation and removal of much of the plasma. The resulting RBC unit has a hematocrit of 0.70-0.80 (70-80%) and a significantly smaller total volume (~200 mL) than the original Whole Blood unit (~450 mL). AS-RBCs are made from units of Whole Blood from which most of the plasma is removed and replaced with 100 mL of a crystalloid (additive) solution. AS-RBCs usually contain a volume of about 300 mL with a hematocrit of about 0.55-0.60 (55-60%). Whole Blood in CPD or CPDA-1 has a hematocrit of approximately 0.38 (38%). Although AS-RBC units have more crystalloid additive solution, units of RBCs and AS-RBCs contain *the same* red cell mass. AS-RBCs are especially useful for anemic patients who cannot tolerate or do not need the blood volume expansion associated with transfusion of Whole Blood units. Clearly, however, fluid overload following transfusion of RBC/AS-RBC units is also possible and remains a medical concern.

Leukocyte-Reduced Red Blood Cells or Leukocyte-Reduced Platelet Concentrates

Patients who have received frequent transfusions or multiparous women who have developed antibodies to HLA and/or white blood cell antigens are candidates for Leukocyte-Reduced Red Blood Cells (LR-RBCs) or Leukocyte-Reduced Platelet Concentrates (LR-PCs).[13,14] Various methods are employed to remove white cells from RBC units or platelet concentrates in order to decrease the frequency of febrile transfusion reactions. According to AABB *Standards for Blood Banks and Transfusion Services,* to be considered leukocyte-reduced, RBC units must be prepared by a method known to retain at least 80% of the original red cells with the final number of residual leukocytes $<5 \times 10^8$ for prevention of febrile transfusion reactions and $<5 \times 10^6$ when intended for other purposes (presumably to prevent HLA alloimmunization or cytomegalovirus transmission).[6] Most experts recommend use of LR-RBCs only after the patient has had two or more febrile reactions. Menitove et al[15] showed that only 15% of patients who experienced nonhemolytic febrile reactions had a similar episode with the next blood transfusion. Despite the relatively infrequent occurrence of febrile transfusion reactions, use of LR-RBCs or LR-PCs in a home transfusion program will ensure that febrile reactions occur rarely. Although leukocyte reduction filters are expensive, they may be cost-effective in a home infusion program.[19,20] They will not, however, prevent allergic reactions (see below). Patients with recurrent serious febrile transfusion reactions should not be maintained in a home transfusion program.

Washed Red Blood Cells

Mild allergic transfusion reactions are manifest as hives and/or a pruritic macular rash. Serious allergic reactions are associated with vasomotor instability, pulmonary compromise or acute onset cardiovascular impairment. Saline-washed RBCs may be used to decrease the frequency of mild allergic (urticarial) reactions. For patients who are IgA-deficient and who have IgG, anti-IgA antibodies,[16] several plasma-removal washing cycles may be needed to ensure a sufficiently low level of antibody in any infused red cell or platelet component. Any fresh frozen plasma (FFP) infused to such patients must be from an IgA-deficient donor. Despite the infrequent occurrence of serious allergic transfusion reactions, use of washed cells in a home transfusion program will further ensure that allergic reactions occur rarely. If a patient continues to have allergic reactions despite use of routinely washed cells, frozen-thawed-deglycerolized RBCs may be effective. These units contain a lower amount of white cells and plasma proteins than washed RBCs. Because preparation occurs in an open system, however, washed or deglycerolized units must be used within 24 hours. If allergic transfusion reactions are of concern for a patient in a home transfusion program, use of standard saline-washed RBCs is acceptable; frozen deglycerolized RBCs are too expensive to recommend for routine use. Patients with recurrent serious allergic transfusion reactions should not be transfused in a home transfusion program.

Fresh Frozen Plasma

FFP is prepared from whole blood by separating and freezing the plasma within 8 hours of phlebotomy. FFP is indicated primarily for replacement of coagulation factors.[21,22] To ensure maintenance of adequate levels of all the coagulation factors during storage, plasma must be stored frozen. FFP is thawed between 30-37 C with constant agitation and should be transfused as soon as possible. It must be used within 24 hours of thawing to obtain maximal levels of labile coagulation factors. Indications for use of FFP in a home transfusion program are extremely limited because most apply to patients requiring coagulation factor replacement; such patients usually need intensive medical care. For example, patients who are bleeding due to multiple coagulation factor deficiencies secondary to liver disease, disseminated intravascular coagulopathy (DIC) or massive transfusion are best treated in a hospital. Those patients with congenital factor deficiencies for which there is no available coagulation concentrate (such as Factor V or XI) may require FFP. Individuals with mild congenital or acquired factor deficiencies including Factor VIII or Factor IX deficiency (hemophilia A or B, respectively) are best treated with commercially available, virus-attenuated concentrates.

Although the indications for transfusion of FFP electively at home are few, some clinical scenarios could probably be agreed upon as being acceptable. Clearly, however, the program's medical director must bear in mind whether the transfusion request is justified. The posttransfusion increment in coagulation factor levels is limited by the low coagulation factor concentration in FFP (1 unit/mL) and the danger of fluid overload. The success of the FFP transfusion should be determined by measuring the individual's prothrombin time, partial thromboplastin time or specific factor levels after infusion. Although logistically difficult, if one is to use FFP in a chronic home transfusion program, personnel should be available to obtain posttransfusion blood samples at the necessary time intervals. Communication among the blood bank, physician, nurse and patient is of paramount importance in deciding on dosage and frequency of FFP administration.

Giving two or three units of FFP without ever evaluating the patient's response is not acceptable medical practice.

Platelets

Platelets are available as random-donor pooled, and random-donor or HLA-matched single-donor components. Random-donor/pooled platelet concentrates are prepared from individual units of Whole Blood; each bag should contain at least 5.5×10^{10} platelets. One unit of random-donor or HLA-matched single-donor platelet concentrates contains at least 3.0×10^{11} platelets in about 200 mL of plasma. This is equivalent to about six units of random-donor platelet concentrates. To decide if platelet transfusions are indicated, the clinical condition of the patient, the platelet count, the cause of the thrombocytopenia and the platelet functional status must be evaluated.[23] While platelet transfusions may not be effective in sustaining an elevated platelet count in patients with rapid platelet destruction (eg, immune thrombocytopenic purpura, DIC), platelet transfusions generally elevate platelet counts in patients with thrombocytopenia secondary to radiation- or chemotherapy-induced bone marrow hypoplasia. Patients with drug-induced thrombocytopenia and functional platelet abnormalities may also require platelet transfusions. Generally, there is little risk of serious bleeding in these patients when the platelet count is above 20×10^9/L (20,000/μL).[22,24-26] Home platelet transfusion therapy would seem most appropriate for individuals who are thrombocytopenic due to chronic or acute malignant conditions. Elderly, nonambulatory patients would benefit from the availability of in-home platelet transfusion; pediatric oncology patients may also be more comfortable receiving platelets at home. The usual dose of random-donor platelets is six to eight units in an adult (1 unit/10 kg body weight) and one or more units in a pediatric patient (0.1 unit/kg body weight). Each random-donor unit contains about 50 mL of plasma. One-hour posttransfusion platelet count increments are useful to assess alloimmunization status, and should not be difficult to obtain as the nurse can draw a CBC before she/he leaves the home.[26,27]

Granulocytes

This component is prepared by centrifugation leukapheresis of a single donor. All of the following indications should be met before granulocyte concentrates are given: 1) bone marrow showing myeloid hypoplasia; 2) neutropenia (<500 polymorphonuclear cells/μL); 3) fever or infection unresponsive to appropriate antibiotic therapy for 24-48 hours; 4) patient with a reasonable chance for survival. A patient with these indications usually requires hospitalization and, therefore, home transfusion of this component is generally inappropriate. The frequency of febrile reactions with granulocyte transfusion is high and this further makes its use in a home transfusion setting undesirable. A terminally ill patient spending any remaining time at home, even if septic and granulocytopenic, is *not* a candidate for home granulocyte transfusion. If antibiotics are discontinued and a "DNR" (do not resuscitate) order is in effect, a volunteer donor should not be recruited to spend 2-3 hours undergoing leukapheresis.

The use of granulocytes in a home infusion program is almost indefensible except, perhaps, for treatment of a patient with a chronic infection who has dysfunctional granulocytes (eg, a patient with chronic granulomatous disease). The risk of serious febrile/hypotensive transfusion reactions is substantial in individuals receiving granulocyte transfusion therapy.

Single-Donor Cryoprecipitate

Cryoprecipitate is prepared by thawing one unit of FFP at 4 C. After thawing, a white precipitate is formed, which is refrozen at –18 C or lower and has a shelf life of 1 year. Each bag of cryoprecipitate contains approximately 80-120 units of Factor VIII:C, about 250 mg of fibrinogen and about 20-30% of the Factor XIII present in the initial unit.[28,29] In addition, approximately 40-70% of the von Willebrand factor present in the initial unit of FFP is recovered in the cryoprecipitate. Before infusion, cryoprecipitate is thawed at 37 C. Cryoprecipitate should be used as soon as possible after thawing. Cryoprecipitate may be used in a home transfusion setting as part of a program of prophylaxis or therapy for von Willebrand's disease. Few, if any, other indications are accepted for use of cryoprecipitate in the home.

Lyophilized Factor Concentrates

Hemophiliacs with moderate to severe congenital Factor VIII deficiency require Factor VIII concentrate. This component is prepared by commercial fractionation and lyophilization of pooled FFP. The concentrates currently available are virus-attenuated by heating, exposure to solvent/detergent, monoclonal purification or a combination of these methods.[30,31] Recombinant forms of Factor VIII are also available.[32] Factor IX concentrates currently on the market are also virus-attenuated. Anti-inhibitor coagulation complex contains Factor VIII inhibitor bypassing activity[33-35] and is indicated for patients with a high titer Factor VIII inhibitor (10-20% of patients with hemophilia A develop a detectable inhibitor to Factor VIII). These blood derivatives have been used by hemophiliacs for home transfusion for many years. In addition to reduced hospitalization, improved psychological outlook and greater social integration have resulted. Current concentrates appear to prevent transmission of lipid-enveloped transfusion-transmitted viruses including HIV-1/2, HTLV-I/II, and hepatitis B and C, but not non-lipid-enveloped viruses such as hepatitis A or parvovirus B19.[36]

Albumin and Plasma Protein Fraction

Albumin is composed of approximately 96% albumin and 4% alpha and beta globulins; Plasma Protein Fraction (PPF) is 86% albumin. These products are indicated for patients who are both hypovolemic and hypoproteinemic.[37,38] Albumin infusion is rarely indicated in a home transfusion program. Use of albumin and a diuretic to treat fluid overload is better performed in a hospital. Hypovolemic, hypotensive patients should receive albumin or other therapy in a hospital, too. Compared to blood or plasma, albumin has a very low incidence of febrile or allergic reactions.

Immune Serum Globulin

Immune Serum Globulin (ISG) is a concentrated aqueous solution of gamma globulin made from pools of human plasma. The intramuscular form is prepared by cold ethanol fractionation. Although IgG is the principal immunoglobulin present, IgA and IgM may also be present. ISG should not be given to patients with IgG, anti-IgA antibodies, especially in a home transfusion setting. The standard ISG preparation is intended for intramuscular injection because the aggregated IgG molecules in the preparation can activate complement via the alternative pathway and produce anaphylactic shock if given intravenously. ISG suitable for intravenous use as replacement therapy for patients with congenital or acquired immunoglobulin deficiency is prepared by a different technique and is useful in the home transfusion setting. Although IVIgG is prepared by a different technique, like its intramuscular counterpart, IVIgG has side effects such as malaise, headache, fever, nausea and tachycardia, which tend to be rate- and dose-related.

Administration of Blood Components

General Considerations

A protocol must be developed for obtaining properly labeled blood samples for typing and crossmatching before transfusion and for ensuring positive patient identification in the home, such as by use of wristbands. A mechanism for transporting the blood component to the home must also be provided. RBCs must be kept between 1-10 C. A portable insulated cooler packed with wet ice such as is used to carry beverages to picnics can be used to transport units of blood or store aliquots of blood not being transfused. RBCs should *never* be placed in a home food refrigerator or freezer because of the danger of hemolysis due to an improper storage temperature as well as the risk of spreading transfusion-transmitted diseases to members of the family. Platelets and thawed FFP are stored at room temperature and can be kept in an empty insulated cooler to avoid extremes of heat or cold. A responsible adult family member should be present at all times.

The rate of administration is initially determined by the physician, but should be modified if medically necessary by the nurse in charge of the transfusion. To ensure accurate records, the nurse should carefully chart patient intake and output. Blood should never be transfused too rapidly or, for that matter, too slowly. Appropriate administration of blood products is critical, especially in a home transfusion setting. Any misunderstanding on the part of the nurse could not only jeopardize the patient's safety but also place that nurse and possibly other medical personnel involved in the home transfusion program at risk of a medical malpractice suit.

Transfusion of over two units of blood or excessive amounts of plasma-containing products could place the patient at great risk of fluid overload and acute pulmonary edema. Acutely ill patients in need of large-volume transfusions should not be transfused in a home setting. Home transfusion is intended to treat chronic anemias, not life-threatening hemorrhage. If over two units of blood are needed for anemic, chronically ill patients, they should be spread out over several days with judicious use of diuretics as necessary to maintain fluid balance. Again, if the fluid balance for such patients is difficult to manage, transfusion should be performed in a hospital setting.

Generally, the number of units of blood or components to be transfused to a patient at home in a day should not exceed either two units of RBCs, 10 units of pooled platelet concentrates, one or two single-donor platelet apheresis products or three units of FFP. All of these are equal to about 500-600 mL of fluid. Most patients who would need more than this amount would likely be critically ill and should be hospitalized.

Each unit of blood or component must be transfused within 4 hours.[7,8] If blood must be transfused in less than 2 hours (eg, to support blood pressure), the patient is too acutely ill and should be transferred to a hospital. Transfusions lasting over 4 hours increase the risk of bacterial growth in the component and fail to comply with established guidelines.[8]

For adult patients with chronic thrombocytopenia due to disease or chemotherapy, 4-10 units of pooled platelet concentrates are suitable for transfusion at one time. Patients requiring massive numbers of platelet transfusions in a desperate attempt to combat hemorrhage should not be transfused in a home setting. Once pooled, platelets must be infused in less than 4 hours. Eight units of pooled platelet concentrates contain 400 mL of plasma (50 mL/bag) and this should be considered in calculating fluid volumes to avoid hypervolemia. All blood components must be transfused through an appropriate filter.

Infusion Pumps

Blood components, including platelets and plasma, can be transfused through electromechanical infusion pumps, if desired. Platelets thus transfused have a normal in-vivo survival.[39] Such pumps, however, may cause hemolysis when used to transfuse high hematocrit RBC products, and dilution of the RBCs with 0.9% NaCl may be necessary, assuming the patient can tolerate the added fluid. AS-RBCs have a lower hematocrit and do not need dilution with saline. In all cases, the infusion pump manufacturer should be consulted to determine the appropriateness of use of that particular device for the transfusion of RBCs. Generally, use of infusion pumps is not necessary. However, they may be useful for pediatric home transfusion.

Blood Warmers

Blood or components must never be heated above 38 C due to the risk of hemolysis. Blood and components do not usually need to be warmed because two units of refrigerated blood will not affect cardiac nerve conduction. Rapid transfusion of multiple units of 4 C blood, however, can induce ventricular arrhythmias.[40] This should not be a concern for home transfusion because no more than two units of blood should be transfused at one time. If blood warming is desired for patient comfort, only an approved electric blood warmer should be used. Never warm blood in tap water. Also, blood *MUST NEVER* be put in a microwave oven. Overheated blood or components can cause hemolysis and/or protein precipitation, which may lead to a fatal transfusion reaction.[41]

Posttransfusion Follow-Up

A method must be available for evaluating posttransfusion changes in hematocrit, platelet count or coagulation factor levels, depending on the blood product transfused. Follow-up usually occurs the day after transfusion. One should not transfuse a patient if no posttransfusion follow-up is planned at all. Good medical practice requires that the results of the transfusion be assessed to determine the efficacy of the therapy as well as the need for future transfusions.

Disposal of Blood Products

A major concern for home transfusion programs relates to the safe disposal of transfusion materials such as empty blood bags, IV tubing, blood-soaked gauzes and, of course, needles and other sharps. The nurse must be very careful to avoid spreading transfusion-transmitted disease via exposure of nonmedical personnel or family members to dirty needles; sanitation workers are also at great potential risk. In addition, disposal of unsterilized blood bags into landfills may be a violation of city or state health codes. Blood bags and other disposables used for the transfusion may need to be autoclaved, incinerated or treated with bleach in order to render them noninfectious; local or state health authorities should be consulted. Clearly, the best method of disposing of these blood products is for the nurse to collect all transfusion-related disposables, especially sharps and needles, in a suitable container and bring them back to the hospital for appropriate disposal; this process should be documented in detailed SOPs. Close monitoring of this area will avoid many health and possibly legal risks that are associated with home transfusion. An empty blood bag, with the hospital's identifying label, found lying in the street could be a health hazard and possibly result in a public relations and legal nightmare.

Premedication

Although most patients who receive transfusions do not experience acute adverse transfusion reactions, those who do must be appropriately treated and the use of a home transfusion setting complicates this process. The concept of prophylactic premedication should be considered. Some physicians feel that it is appropriate that patients with, or even without, a history of previous febrile or allergic reactions receive an antihistamine or an antipyretic before transfusion. Other physicians feel that LR-RBCs or LR-PCs should be used routinely for home transfusions because this practice could eliminate the need for premedication as well as significantly reduce the incidence of febrile nonhemolytic transfusion reactions. Use of leukocyte-reduced components is preferable to the use of premedication with non-leukocyte-reduced units of blood because filtration is more effective than pharmacotherapy in decreasing the incidence of febrile reactions. The use of antipyretics such as acetaminophen (or aspirin in nonthrombocytopenic patients) will blunt, but not eliminate, significant febrile reactions. Allergic transfusion reactions may respond to oral or intravenous administration of 25-50 mg of diphenhydramine. In adults, 100 mg of hydrocortisone IV or 25 mg of meperidine administered subcutaneously or intramuscularly can stop severe chills. Although cost is a consideration, medical as well as legal concerns should prompt in-home use of the component that is least likely to provoke a transfusion reaction. Thus, leukocyte-reduced or washed RBCs are to be strongly considered for use in home transfusion settings. Leukocyte-reduction blood filters will not prevent allergic reactions. Washing platelets is not feasible in most situations, and is indicated primarily for patients with IgG, anti-IgA antibodies. Platelet washing protocols have been published.[42] Again, patients with a prior history of repetitive and/or severe transfusion reactions should not be transfused at home.

Transfusion Reactions

It is widely accepted that any transfusion carries with it a risk to the patient. Each patient should be carefully monitored during and after transfusion for any adverse signs or symptoms.[12] These may include acute problems such as hemolysis, fever, chills, hives or congestive heart failure. Delayed reactions include hemolysis and transmission of infectious diseases such as hepatitis or cytomegalovirus. This section addresses both hemolytic and nonhemolytic transfusion reactions, which may be either immediate or delayed in their mode of presentation.[43,44]

Hemolytic Transfusion Reactions

Acute hemolytic reactions are caused by high titer and/or high avidity antibodies in the recipient's plasma, which destroy the donor's red cells. Hemolysis may be either intravascular (almost always from ABO incompatibility) or extravascular (anti-K, anti-D, anti-Fy^a, etc). Acute intravascular hemolytic reactions can be fatal. The clinical signs include hemoglobinuria and hemoglobinemia. Among the more important clinical symptoms are fever, chills, back pain and possibly shock. Activation of the complement and coagulation cascade can result in cardiorespiratory collapse or DIC, respectively. If the concentration of antibodies is insufficient in the recipient at the time of transfusion of incompatible blood, no adverse reactions may occur acutely. However, subsequent synthesis of antibody may result in hemolysis of the circulating donor blood cells 7-10 days after transfusion (delayed hemolytic transfusion reaction). In contrast to a life-threatening acute intravascular hemolytic reaction, delayed extravascular reactions may be clinically inapparent. The only manifestation of a delayed extravascular reaction may be a decrease in hematocrit. Proper patient follow-up and comprehensive blood bank records are required to evaluate these types of reactions. Almost all acute hemolytic reactions are caused by clerical errors resulting in the wrong blood being transfused to the wrong patient; only rarely are blood bank technical errors responsible.[45] It is mandatory that a system for positive patient identification be provided to ensure that the blood and the patient are both properly identified before transfusion, especially in the home setting. An individual who can identify the recipient must be present.

Febrile Transfusion Reactions

Fever is common to both hemolytic and nonhemolytic transfusion reactions. Febrile, nonhemolytic transfusion reactions are characterized by chills followed by a rise in temperature to over 101 F. These reactions usually occur within the first 1-3 hours of transfusion and are due to leukoagglutinin or cytotoxic antibodies. The role of cytokines, such as IL-1, IL-6, IL-8 or TNF-α, is now being recognized as causing many of the clinical symptoms seen in patients with febrile transfusion reactions.[46-49] Most patients with febrile reactions will respond favorably to aspirin (if medically permitted for the nonthrombocytopenic patient) or acetaminophen; symptoms usually abate in 4-6 hours. Due to the inflammatory component, febrile reactions can also presage a hemolytic transfusion reaction. Thus, fever and chills must be viewed as potentially serious until hemolysis can be ruled out by evaluation of the patient's urine or plasma. A fever or chill during transfusion should result in immediate cessation of the infusion. The decision to transfuse any additional blood components should be made after consultation with the patient's physician and the blood bank physician.

Septic transfusion reactions are often fatal and may also present as fever and chills. These types of reactions are more commonly seen with transfusion of units of platelet concentrates that are stored at 20-24 C. Patients who receive a unit of bacterially contaminated blood develop fever and chills, which may progress rapidly to shock and cardiac arrest.[50] Units of contaminated blood almost always appear normal without any associated strange odors, discoloration or gas bubbles. Therapy following transfusion of a contaminated unit of blood includes immediate support of blood pressure, maintenance of airway patency and emergent use of antibiotics. Clearly, infusion of a unit of contaminated blood in a hospital or home transfusion setting can be a medical disaster. If such a complication occurs in a home transfusion setting, the patient should be immediately transported to a tertiary-care hospital.

Allergic Reactions

Allergic reactions consist of hives and itching, which usually develop during the blood transfusion. The reaction may be limited to the site of transfusion or generalized to the face, trunk and extremities. It is believed that antibodies against plasma proteins are responsible. Most reactions are mild and respond to antihistamines.

Epinephrine and steroids may be used for more severe symptoms involving bronchospasm. Severe allergic reactions can be life-threatening. In Vyas's series,[51] 86% of subjects who had anaphylactic or anaphylactoid transfusion reactions had anti-IgA antibodies. Thus, patients who have a history of severe allergic or anaphylactic transfusion reactions should be evaluated for such antibodies. Washed RBCs and IgA-deficient plasma can be used for future transfusions in such patients.[52] IgA-deficient patients with a history of anaphylactic reactions and patients with a history of other severe allergic reactions should not be transfused at home.

Evaluation of Suspected Transfusion Reactions

When a transfusion reaction is suspected, the blood infusion must be stopped at once and the remaining component, together with a posttransfusion blood sample from the patient, must be returned to the blood bank. There, testing will be done in order to exclude a hemolytic transfusion reaction or clerical errors. Such patients should be evaluated by a physician so that appropriate decisions regarding therapy can be made. In the home transfusion setting, however, such evaluation may be appropriately performed over the phone if the on-site (ie, in the patient's home) health-care worker can appropriately convey the clinical situation to the physician. Rapid communication between the home health-care worker and the responsible physician is crucial so that appropriate steps may be taken.

Conclusion

Transfusion of blood outside the hospital setting is fraught with dangers. If the hospital transfusion service wishes to provide blood, it should ensure that the blood is appropriately used because the hospital will likely be held ultimately responsible for what occurs. All aspects of an out-of-hospital transfusion program should be detailed in the institution's SOPs, including the following:

- Selection of suitable patients
- Patient identification
- Indications for the transfusion of various components
- Proper blood administration
- Monitoring of the nursing staff
- Blood administration (including quantity of blood, flow rates, whether blood can be infused with other medications)

- Storage conditions such as Igloos® or refrigerators
- Use of infusion pumps or blood warmers
- Posttransfusion follow-up
- Disposal of blood products and return of any blood, needles, sharps, gauze, etc
- Patient premedication
- What emergency precautions should be taken
- What medications can be given
- Whether nurses can intubate
- Ambulance availability
- Physician availability
- Notification and work-up of transfusion reactions

Transfusion in a clinic can be considered to be an extension of the hospital. In that sense, all appropriate hospital concerns must be met. The identification and work-up of hemolytic, febrile and allergic reactions in the outpatient setting must be frequently reviewed. A periodic review of quality assurance/quality control issues is necessary.

As with all aspects of medicine, if we do not get our own house in order, the legislative and legal communities will do it for us. It is foolish to set up a home transfusion system that functions on a "no frills" basis. Home transfusion is sound from medical, patient care and economic perspectives. However, it must emphasized that convenience, expediency and financial savings are never placed over the primary concerns for patient health and safety. In this way, home transfusion therapy can take its place as an acceptable form of hemotherapy.

References

1. DePalma L, Snyder EL. Medical aspects of transfusion therapy. In: Snyder EL, Menitove JE, eds. Home transfusion therapy. Arlington, VA: American Association of Blood Banks, 1986:25-40.
2. Beck ML, Grindon AJ. Home transfusion therapy. Transfusion 1986;26:296-7.
3. Miller PC. Home blood component therapy, an alternative. Cambridge: National Intravenous Therapy Association, 1986; 3:213-17.
4. AMA Council on Scientific Affairs. Home care in the 1990s. JAMA 1990;263:1241-4.
5. Pluth NM, ed. A home care transfusion program. Oncology Nurses Forum 1987;14:43-6.

6. Klein H, ed. Standards for blood banks and transfusion services. 16th ed. Bethesda, MD: American Association of Blood Banks, 1994.
7. Pisciotto P, ed. Blood transfusion therapy: A physician's handbook. 4th ed. Bethesda, MD: American Association of Blood Banks, 1993.
8. Circular of information for the use of human blood and blood components, American Association of Blood Banks, American Red Cross, Council of Community Blood Centers, 1993 (revised periodically).
9. Silberstein L, ed. Out-of-hospital transfusions. Bethesda, MD: American Association of Blood Banks, 1992.
10. Crocker KS, Coker MH. Initiation of a home hemotherapy program using a primary nursing model. J Intraven Nurs 1990; 13:13-19.
11. Rutman R, Kakaiya R, Miller WV. Home transfusion for the cancer patient. Semin Oncol Nursing 1990;6:163-7.
12. Snyder EL. Transfusion reactions. In: Benz EJ, Cohen HJ, Furie B, et al, eds. Hematology—Basic principles and practice. New York: Churchill Livingstone, 1991:1644-51.
13. Milner LV, Butcher K. Transfusion reactions reported after transfusions of red blood cells and of whole blood. Transfusion 1978;18:493-5.
14. Thulstrup H. The influence of leukocyte and thrombocyte incompatibility on non-haemolytic transfusion reactions. Vox Sang 1971;21:233-50.
15. Menitove JE, McElligott MC, Aster RH. Febrile transfusion reactions: What blood component should be given next? Vox Sang 1982;42:318-21.
16. Goldfinger D, Lowe C. Prevention of adverse reactions to blood transfusion by the administration of saline-washed red blood cells. Transfusion 1981;21:277-80.
17. Wenz B, Gurtlinger KF, O'Toole AM, Dugan EP. The preparation of granulocyte poor red blood cells by microaggregate filtration. Vox Sang 1980;39:282-7.
18. Schned AR, Silver H. The use of microaggregate filtration in the prevention of febrile transfusion reactions. Transfusion 1981;21:675-81.
19. Snyder EL. Clinical role of leukocyte-depleted blood components. Transfusion 1989;29:568-71.
20. Lane TA, Anderson KC, Goodnough LT, et al. Leukocyte reduction in blood component therapy. Ann Intern Med 1992;117: 151-62.

21. NIH Consensus Conference. Fresh frozen plasma—Indications and risks. JAMA 1985;253:551-3.
22. National Blood Resource Education Program Expert Panel. Transfusion alert—Indications for the use of red blood cells, platelets, and fresh frozen plasma. Bethesda, MD: National Heart, Lung, and Blood Institute, 1993. NIH Publication No. 93-2974a.
23. Slichter SJ. Controversies in platelet transfusion therapy. Annu Rev Med 1980;31:509-40.
24. Gaydos LA, Freireich EJ, Mantel N. The quantitative relationship between platelet count and hemorrhage in patients with acute leukemia. N Engl J Med 1962;266:905-9.
25. Slichter SJ, Harker LA. Thrombocytopenia: Mechanisms and management of defects in platelet production. Clin Haematol 1978;7:523-39.
26. Daly PA, Schiffer CA, Aisner J, Wiernick PH. Platelet transfusion therapy—One hour posttransfusion increments are valuable in predicting the need for HLA-matched preparations. JAMA 1980;243:435-8.
27. O'Connell B, Lee EJ, Schiffer CA. The value of 10 minute post-transfusion platelet counts. Transfusion 1988;28:66-7.
28. Ness PM, Perkins HA. Cryoprecipitate as a reliable source of fibrinogen replacement. JAMA 1979;241:1690-1.
29. Kitchens CS, Newcomb TF. Factor XIII. Medicine 1979;58:413-29.
30. Horowitz B, Wiebe M, Lippin A, Strycker MH. Inactivation of viruses in labile blood derivatives. I. Disruption of lipid-enveloped viruses by tri(n-butyl)phosphate detergent combinations. Transfusion 1986;25:516-22.
31. Tocci LJ, Napychank PA, Cable RG, Snyder EL. The effect of solvent/detergent-treated plasma on stored platelet concentrates. Transfusion 1993;33:145-9.
32. Schwartz RS, Abildgaard CF, Aledort LM, et al. Human recombinant DNA-derived antihemophilic factor (Factor VIII) in the treatment of hemophilia A. N Engl J Med 1990;323:1800-5.
33. Hilgartner MW, Knatterud GL, FEIBA Study Group. The use of factor eight inhibitor bypassing activity (FEIBA IMMUNO) product for treatment of bleeding episodes in hemophiliacs with inhibitors. Blood 1982;61:36-40.
34. Abildgaard CP, Penner JA, Watson-Williams J. Anti-inhibitor coagulant complex (Autoplex) for treatment of factor VIII inhibitors in hemophilia. Blood 1980;56:978-84.

35. Lusher JM, Shapiro SS, Palascak JE, et al. Efficacy of prothrombin complex concentrates in hemophiliacs with antibodies to factor VIII. N Engl J Med 1980;303:421-5.
36. Mannucci PM, Gdovin S, Gringeri A, et al. Transmission of hepatitis A to patients with hemophilia by factor VIII concentrates treated with organic solvent and detergent to inactivate viruses. Ann Intern Med 1994;120:1-7.
37. Tullis JL. Albumin 2. Guidelines for clinical use. JAMA 1977; 237:460-3.
38. Snyder E. Clinical use of albumin, plasma protein fraction and isoimmune globulin products. In: Silvergleid A, Britten A, eds. Plasma products: Use and management. Arlington, VA: American Association of Blood Banks, 1982:87-107.
39. Snyder EL, Ferri PM, Smith EO, Ezekowitz MD. Use of an electromechanical infusion pump for transfusion of platelet concentrates. Transfusion 1984;24:524-7.
40. Boyan CP, Howland WE. Cardiac arrest and temperature of bank blood. JAMA 1963;183:58-61.
41. Arens JF, Leonard GL. Danger of overwarming blood by microwave. JAMA 1971;218:1045-6.
42. Kalman ND, Brown DJ. Platelet washing with a blood cell processor. Transfusion 1982;22:125-7.
43. Solauki C, McCurdy PR. Delayed hemolytic transfusion reactions. An often-missed entity. JAMA 1978;239:729.
44. Pineda AA, Brzica SM, Taswell HF. Hemolytic transfusion reaction: Recent experience in a large blood bank. Mayo Clin Proc 1978;53:378-90.
45. Honig CL, Bove JR. Transfusion-associated fatalities: A review of Bureau of Biologics reports 1976-1978. Transfusion 1980; 20:653-61.
46. Stack G, Snyder EL. Cytokine generation in stored platelet concentrates. Transfusion 1994;34:20-5.
47. Muylle L, Joos M, Wouters E, et al. Increased tumor necrosis factor-α (TNF-α), interleukin 1 (IL-1) and interleukin 6 (IL-6) levels in the plasma of stored platelet concentrates: Relationship between TNF-a and IL-6 levels and febrile transfusion reactions. Transfusion 1993;33:195-9.
48. Dinarello CA. Interleukin-1 and interleukin-1 antagonism. Blood 1991;77:1627-52.
49. Davenport RD, Strieter RM, Standiford TJ, Kunkel SL. Interleukin-8 production in red blood cell incompatibility. Blood 1990;76:2439-42.

50. Goldman M, Blajchman MA. Blood product-associated bacterial sepsis. Transfus Med Rev 1991;5:73-83.
51. Vyas GN, Holmdahl L, Perkins HA, Fudenberg HH. Serological specificity of human anti-IgA and its significance in transfusion. Blood 1969;34:573.
52. Yap PL, Pryde EAD, McClelland DBL. IgA content of frozen-thawed-washed red blood cells and blood products measured by radioimmunoassay. Transfusion 1982;22:36-8.

In: Fridey JL, Kasprisin CA and Issitt LA, eds.
Out-of-Hospital Transfusion Therapy
Bethesda, MD: American Association of Blood Banks, 1994

2

Out-of-Hospital Transfusion: A Regional Blood Center Approach

Cherie S. Evans, MD

THE DELIVERY OF COMPLEX medical care, including blood transfusion, in nonhospital settings is not new. As early as 1970, there were published reports of successful home transfusion programs for hemophiliacs.[1] Given the psychological trauma induced by hospitalization in a patient population composed largely of children, the benefits outweighed the potential risk. However, concerns about the liability involved in such care continued to hamper a wider acceptance of the practice.[2] With the increasing demand for health-care cost containment, beginning in the 1980s and accelerating in the 1990s, many health-care providers began to reassess the need for such a conservative approach to a wide variety of highly complex forms of medical care including those with possible adverse outcomes such as transfusion. Recently, a presidential commission reevaluated our entire system of health care in order to identify mechanisms of cost containment as a matter of the highest national urgency. Reducing dependence on expensive hospital-based care is clearly a part of this evolving plan.

The advent of the AIDS epidemic spotlighted the need for more flexible out-of-hospital care for this growing population of patients requiring repetitive and often lengthy hospitalizations. Studies of efforts in New York City and San Francisco to cope with the demands on health-care resources due to AIDS make a strong case for expanded nonhospital care on both a humane basis and an economic one.[3,4] Multitransfused patients are also likely to be receiving at home other traditionally hospital-based and complicated therapies

Cherie S. Evans, MD, Medical Director, Blood Bank of the Alameda-Contra Costa Medical Association, Oakland, California such as intravenous chemotherapy and parenteral nutrition, making a refusal to provide transfusion in the same setting untenable and unsupportable.

Other changes in the patient population are fueling the fire. There is an ever-increasing elderly patient population for whom physical mobility is often a problem. This population is likely to have conditions requiring chronic care and to be less affluent and living on fixed incomes, all indications for non-hospital-based care whenever possible.[5] With the growth of health-care consumerism, greater patient involvement in and responsibility for health-care choices are being demanded. It has even been suggested that this may be "the most important trend in health care in the final quarter of this century."[6] Invariably, when patients are given the option, therapy provided outside the hospital is preferred.

In response to this demand, an increasing number of highly sophisticated outpatient health-care delivery systems have been developed to provide a wide array of high technology medical care. This includes modalities such as hemodialysis, parenteral nutrition and infusion therapies such as cancer chemotherapy, antibiotics, pain control, gamma globulin, α_1-antitrypsin and pentamidine. Although these forms of care are known to be associated with significant risks including such potentially fatal complications as anaphylaxis, it has become the standard of care nationwide to provide such care in nonhospital settings, even in the home.

Several organizational approaches to out-of-hospital transfusion have been developed. Many hospital-based transfusion services have extended their scope of practice and are providing crossmatching and nursing services in a variety of outpatient settings. Although in 1986 some felt it unlikely that blood centers would become significantly involved in outpatient transfusion,[7] in California it has become common for regional blood centers to provide transfusion services for nonhospital facilities. Advantages and disadvantages to each approach are outlined in Table 2-1. This chapter describes the regional blood center approach.

Quality Assurance

Quality assurance (QA) is one of the most important issues to be addressed when providing transfusion services.[8] Even though transfusion outside a hospital is increasingly common, it carries a greater risk than hospital transfusion, at least in terms of liability and

Table 2-1. Organizational Approaches to Out-of-Hospital Transfusion Services

I. HOSPITAL-BASED OUT-OF-HOSPITAL TRANSFUSION SERVICES

A. Advantages

1. Mechanism in place for transfusion service quality assurance/assessment
   a. Transfusion committee in existence
   b. Audit criteria already developed
2. Laboratory and nursing personnel may be from same facility
3. Additional income for laboratory

B. Disadvantages

1. Provides transfusion only for patients of physicians on own medical staff
2. Not routinely set up to ship components
3. May not be able to fill special orders internally (cytomegalovirus-negative, irradiated, washed, leukocyte-reduced)

II. REGIONAL-BLOOD-CENTER-BASED TRANSFUSION SERVICE

A. Advantages

1. Centralization: a single set of forms and procedures despite multiple nursing agencies, ordering physicians and hospitals
2. Special orders: equipped to provide special requests on a routine basis
3. Shipping of all components is routine
4. Additional income for laboratory

B. Disadvantages

1. No standing transfusion committee
2. Large time commitment to review procedures of each agency or facility for which blood is provided
3. Quality assurance needs for auditing practice and inspections more difficult to meet

perhaps medically as well. Thus, it is particularly important to establish standard operating procedures (SOPs) that will minimize adverse outcomes, and, in the rare event that any occur, ensure that they will be appropriately handled. In addition, the practice must be audited and monitored over time to detect deviations from approved procedures or unexpected outcomes to determine if they could have been prevented. If such deviations or adverse outcomes occur, a mechanism must be in place to take effective and timely corrective action.

Depending on the structure of the system, QA may be the single most difficult issue for a regional blood center to address. A few centers employ their own blood center nurses to perform the transfusions. These centers take the order for transfusion directly from the patient's attending physician, obtain the patient sample, perform the pretransfusion testing, provide the blood components and perform the transfusion. In such cases, the entire process is centralized and systems for auditing and control of abuse can be patterned after those that have been employed by hospitals since the 1970s and are known to be effective when applied diligently.[9] This situation, however, is the exception.

Most regional centers, whose nurses are not otherwise involved in patient care, choose to provide only the blood components, pretransfusion testing and assistance with reaction evaluation. The blood center develops contractual agreements with outside agencies, such as home nursing infusion services, surgicenters or hemodialysis centers, which receive the order from the attending physician, perform the transfusion, provide for follow-up care for the patient and maintain patient records. Because the "transfusion service" is split between two independent entities, implementation and enforcement of traditional QA mechanisms can be compromised.

Many blood centers address this concern by employing a system of concurrent review of appropriateness of transfusion of any component ordered by the outpatient services. The medical director predetermines acceptable transfusion criteria. A transfusion service request form requires the ordering facility to supply the patient's diagnosis, indication for transfusion and necessary supporting laboratory values obtained within 1 week of the planned transfusion. The blood center's transfusion service SOPs then direct the laboratory technologists to refer any order not meeting predetermined transfusion criteria to the medical director or other designated physician for evaluation before providing blood for the outside facility. If necessary, the ordering physician may need to be consulted to clarify the indication for transfusion and its appropriateness in the outpatient setting, but the final decision to provide the requested components rests with the blood center physician. If indeed transfusion in the outpatient setting poses a risk, this procedure may at least prevent unwarranted transfusion or inappropriate component choices.

Although such procedures ensure an excellent base for a QA program, regional blood centers must also rely on the facilities for which they provide blood to perform their own monitoring of those transfusion aspects that are beyond the control of the blood center.

Therefore, before establishing a contract for outpatient transfusion services, blood centers should require documentation of the facility's QA program. At a minimum, the facility should have a designated medical director, specification of the qualifications required for transfusionists, a plan for continuing education and some mechanism for review of transfusion records and any reactions that occur. Most nursing agencies, particularly those accredited by the Joint Commission on Accreditation of Healthcare Organizations (JCAHO), already have such programs in place for their other home care programs.[10] However, these programs should not be applied directly to their transfusion practice; rather, a program should be designed specifically for blood transfusion. The American Association of Blood Banks guidelines for home transfusion therapy,[11] developed by the Scientific Section Coordinating Committee in 1986, recommended that there be a formal transfusion committee, and an increasing number of home health nursing agencies are following this recommendation. Unfortunately, because most surgicenters, dialysis centers and physicians' offices do not have such protocols and are reluctant to develop them, some blood centers deal only with nursing agencies.

In addition, the blood center must have a mechanism to ensure that its staff will be involved in the evaluation of all adverse transfusion reactions. Although it may not be possible for the blood center to perform the serologic work-up of a reaction, especially if the patient has been transported to a hospital, the center should at least be notified of the reaction and the outcome. Agencies performing home transfusions often require a posttransfusion assessment of outcome both in terms of expected response and evidence of delayed reactions. This assessment is usually done within the first week after the transfusion but, in the case of the elderly for whom volume overload may be a more common unexpected outcome, the assessment might best occur within the first 24 hours. Because posttransfusion assessments are generally not done for transfusions in surgicenters and physicians' offices, it is impossible to determine if delayed reactions are occurring.

One of the most difficult questions has been how the blood center should go about ensuring that outside facilities are actually performing transfusions in accordance with current good medical practice and the policies and procedures originally approved by the blood center medical director. Many blood center medical directors review each agency's policies and standard operating procedures, their contract for biohazardous waste disposal, their continuing education and QA programs and qualifications of transfusionists. Although this can be an extremely time-consuming undertaking, it does at least ensure that the facility staff have sufficient knowledge to present an acceptable program. This does not, however, ensure that the facility will follow its stated plan or that inappropriate practices will not develop over time. Some indicators that would alert the blood center to potential lack of compliance or changes in the outside facility's operation can be tracked. Examples of such indicators are given in Table 2-2. In one blood center, investigation of a sharp increase in inaccurately or incompletely filled out transfusion service request forms revealed that the transfusion agency had lost its transfusion nurse and was temporarily employing nurses from another agency, a practice that was promptly halted once identified. A few blood centers offer to train the transfusionists for the facilities with which they work and to inspect the facilities annually. Others, feeling this active approval of the other facility's program results in increased liability, detail in their contract which QA activities will be the responsibility of the outside facility.

Regardless of the extent to which a blood center chooses to involve itself in the outpatient transfusion service QA program, it must remember that if moral and ethical persuasion fail to obtain compliance from an independent facility, the center's only enforcement mechanism is denial of blood components. Before embarking on such a program or accepting a new facility, consider the implications of denial of blood components. Would there be a local hospital available where the procedure and transfusion could be performed? What if the

Table 2-2. Audit Criteria for Regional Blood Centers

I. ORDERS FOR COMPONENTS

A. Appropriate indication for specific component
B. Correct component chosen
C. Forms filled out completely and accurately

II. RECORDS (POSTTRANSFUSION REPORT RETURNED TO BLOOD CENTER)

A. Complete
B. Legible
C. Accurate
D. Timely

III. EVIDENCE OF INAPPROPRIATE PATIENT SELECTION

IV. OCCURRENCE OF ERRORS BY TRANSFUSION AGENCY PERSONNEL DISCOVERED BY THE BLOOD CENTER

units in question were autologous? What would happen if the services had been prepaid by the patient? What impact would it have on the community's perception of the blood center?

Patient Selection

Another critical element in a successful outpatient transfusion service is appropriate patient selection. Because full hospital emergency services are not immediately available, nonhospital sites are not the setting in which unstable or acutely ill individuals should be transfused. Typically, appropriate patients are those with chronic conditions and stable cardiovascular, respiratory and fluid status for whom transport to the hospital would present a significant physical, financial or psychological problem. Table 2-3 lists typical conditions for which outpatient transfusion is often chosen. To ensure that the patient's condition has not changed, the personal physician should evaluate the patient within the week before the intended transfusion.

In addition to the patient's physical condition, various other circumstances are critical to patient selection. In the unlikely event of a serious transfusion reaction, emergency help must be adequate and rapidly available. In most large urban centers with an adequate rapid emergency response ("911") service, this is not a problem, but an increasing number of rural areas are considering out-of-hospital transfusion as an alternative to transporting patients over tremendous distances to the nearest hospital. In such cases, considerable attention should be given to how a serious reaction would be handled. At a minimum, consultation with a physician must be immediately available, even if only by telephone. In cases in which

Table 2-3. Typical Conditions Treated in Out-of-Hospital Transfusion Setting

1. End-stage renal disease
2. ARC/AIDS
3. Hemoglobinopathy
4. Anemia of chronic disease
5. Myelosclerosis, myelodysplasia, myelophthistic states
6. Chronic bleeding
7. Nonimmune thrombocytopenia
8. Coagulation factor deficiency
9. Autologous transfusion in outpatient surgery setting
10. Hemolytic anemia

physicians will not be present at the facility at the time of the transfusion, some mechanism to ensure physician availability should be in place. One common practice is to have the nurse call the ordering physician immediately before initiating the procedure. It is essential that another competent adult be present during the entire procedure. If there should be a reaction so severe that the nurse is completely occupied with the patient, this individual is then able to call for emergency help and relay information to and instructions from the attending physician.

Some outdated patient selection criteria have appeared in the home transfusion literature and become incorporated into home nursing agency protocols. The first of these is the requirement that the patient must have been transfused previously with a similar component in a hospital setting without an adverse reaction.[12] One immediate life-threatening reaction that could be caused by transfusion is anaphylaxis, which is not unique to blood transfusion. Any facility performing intravenous drug therapy of any kind must have staff competent to handle this reaction. If the concern is for an unexpected acute hemolytic transfusion reaction, then the safest red blood cell transfusion a patient ever receives is the first unless there has been pregnancy-induced alloimmunization. In addition, the likelihood that an alloantibody undetected by a two-cell or three-cell antibody screen will cause a severe or fatal reaction is remote.[13] It seems more reasonable to put extra effort into preventing an accidental ABO mismatch, which can cause a fatal reaction even in a hospital setting. In addition to the necessary clerical checks, one additional step would be to employ a check cell system similar to that used in some hospitals. If a patient is new to the blood center transfusion service, then two samples are drawn and ABO grouped; the first is the sample obtained for the crossmatch and the second is a sample drawn just before picking up the unit(s) for transfusion. Before releasing the unit of blood, the blood center laboratory performs a simple ABO grouping to verify that the ABO group is identical to that recorded for the recipient. Alternatively, some centers choose to give nothing but group O packed cells the first time a patient is transfused through their service. In some surgicenters, where most transfusions are autologous, an identification system is used in which at the time of the donation, the patient is given a coded arm band that corresponds to a code that will open a locked storage bag into which the unit is placed at the time of donation. When the transfusionist wants to use the blood, the code on the arm band is used to open the lock on the storage bag, and is the only code that can open the lock.[14]

The second questionable and unduly conservative selection criterion employed by some agencies is that the patient have no known clinically significant alloantibodies. If the patient has a well-documented transfusion history, uncomplicated serology with clearly delineated alloantibody specificity(ies), and underlying undetected antibodies have been ruled out, then the blood center may select antigen-negative units and crossmatch for compatibility just as a hospital would, and yet place the patient at no greater risk.

Pretransfusion Patient Evaluation

If a transfusion is to occur in a patient's home, then the home itself needs to be evaluated. Is there a phone? Is the home accessible by road if an ambulance is needed? Will there be another responsible adult available? Regardless of the location of the transfusion, the patient's baseline clinical condition must be evaluated and documented in writing. In the home setting, this evaluation is usually done when the blood sample for the crossmatch is obtained. In surgicenters, dialysis centers and physicians' offices, the evaluation is done when the patient presents for the procedure.

As in the hospital, adequate and accurate patient identification is a key element in preventing fatal transfusion reactions. Except for autologous transfusions, this identification process begins during the pretransfusion evaluation. The blood center must ensure that procedures are in place to prevent misidentification of the patient or the blood and that these procedures will be strictly enforced. Because of the well-documented continuing occurrence of fatalities due to simple clerical errors, many services are employing physical means of identification such as the arm bands previously described and even photographs of patients.[15] In addition, at every critical step two separate individuals should check the identification of the patient and the unit, as well as the unit's blood group, outdate and appearance. If at any point there is a discrepancy, even when those involved are convinced it is a simple transcription error, the unit must not be transfused and the pretransfusion procedures should be repeated with appropriate steps to verify identification of patient and unit.

Informed Consent

In states such as California, concerns about consent for routine inpatient transfusion have led to explicit legislation addressing the requirement for and format of the informed consent that is to be obtained in advance of elective surgery that presents the possibility of transfusion.[16] Because out-of-hospital transfusion may pose different risks to the patient than hospital-based care, an informed consent that specifically addresses these issues must be obtained. Although this responsibility ultimately rests with the patient's attending physician, it is prudent for any nursing agency working with such patients to ascertain that the patient has been adequately informed and has no outstanding concerns, and to document that fact in the record.

Compatibility Testing and Component Choice

Compatibility testing for outpatients is not significantly different than that for inpatients. It is not unusual, however, for blood centers to make more conservative choices than would be made for hospitalized patients. For example, although the immediate-spin crossmatch is now commonly used for patients with a negative antibody screen, many outpatient services still employ a full antiglobulin crossmatch. Some centers also routinely perform an autocontrol on the patient with each crossmatch. However, in areas with a large population of recipients with HIV infection or other conditions associated with nonspecific IgG autoantibodies, such a practice may provide little protection and significantly increase costs.

The general indications for choice of component are the same as for hospital practice and are well-delineated elsewhere.[17] A few components are not appropriate in the out-of-hospital transfusion setting; these include whole blood and granulocytes. Patients with an appropriate indication for either of these components are acutely ill and require hospitalization.

Shipping Procedure

Regional blood centers are particularly well-equipped to handle the shipment of all blood components. Centers in compliance with AABB standards and federal regulations will have already validated their shipping procedures as adequate to maintain units at the appropriate temperature for a specific time span. The transfusing agency is required to pick up the units within that time frame and leave the shipping container intact until immediately before transfusion. In addition, some blood centers place temperature-sensitive tags on the units that will change color to indicate if the unit has not remained at the appropriate temperature. Once the shipping container is opened, all of the units it contains must be transfused within the time specified by the SOP. If a multiunit transfusion is expected to require more time than that specified, each of the units should be packed separately. If the transfusion facility plans to transfuse more than one patient in a single day, it may be convenient for them to pick up all the units at the same time. Some blood centers allow this, while others require that each patient's units and identifying paperwork be packed separately. When the shipping container is packed, blood center personnel should document the appearance of the unit(s) and obtain the signature of the person transporting the blood.

Minimizing Risk of Adverse Reactions

As with any transfusion, consideration should be given to anything that can be done to prevent adverse reactions. The cost:benefit ratio may be slightly skewed compared to that observed in hospitals, but somewhat greater cost may be acceptable in view of the potentially greater liability and medical risk. It is often stated that patients should receive no more than two units per 24-hour period when transfused in the home.[18] However, many agencies choose to ensure that the amount transfused per transfusion event is individualized to suit the specific patient's condition. Elderly patients, with more susceptibility to volume overload, may more appropriately be given only one unit per 24-hour period. A young HIV-infected individual with profound anemia, excellent cardiovascular and respiratory reserve and volume depletion due to diarrhea or other conditions may tolerate three or even four units of packed cells a day without any increased risk. Such individualized choices, however, should actively involve the medical director in determining criteria or evaluating individual cases.

Some forms of leukocyte-reduced cellular components are often used in the outpatient setting, if only to prevent febrile nonhemolytic reactions. Simple filtration at the bedside or in the blood center is replacing washing as the method of choice, although some blood centers will use washed units from donors with alloantibodies. Washing will remove most of the plasma, thus, the alloantibody. (This confers an additional advantage because the expiration time of a washed unit ensures that it will be transfused within 24 hours.)

In addition, physicians often premedicate such patients prophylactically with an antihistamine and/or an antipyretic.

Generally speaking, the old advice to "keep it simple" pertains to out-of-hospital transfusion. Blood warmers are unnecessary in this setting. If blood must be given so rapidly that warming is required, the patient belongs in a hospital. Infusion pumps are rarely indicated unless needed to control the rate of transfusion for small children. If a pump is used, it must be approved for use with the blood component being given.

Monitoring Protocol

In many situations, outpatient transfusions are the best monitored transfusions. This is particularly true in the home where one nurse attends one patient during the entire transfusion and for as long as an hour or more after the procedure. In addition to documentation of the baseline and final condition of the patient, vital signs should be monitored frequently during the first 15 minutes of the procedure and then every 30 minutes until the procedure is completed. If any unexplained deviation from baseline occurs, the transfusion should be stopped, the intravenous line kept open with normal saline and the patient evaluated for a possible transfusion reaction. Only rarely and with specific instructions from the attending physician should such a transfusion be restarted.

Posttransfusion Protocol

Patients also need to be educated about the signs and symptoms of delayed transfusion reactions, which may occur when no one with medical training is monitoring them closely. If patients are at home or will be discharged from the outpatient facility immediately after the transfusion, they should be given written instructions about the signs and/or symptoms—and the expected time frame of occurrence—that should prompt them to seek medical attention. These written instructions should provide names and telephone numbers for individuals who would be responsible for answering questions and arranging for emergency care or other medical follow-up if necessary. Ideally, a medical professional should make an appointment to personally reevaluate the patient at some time within the first week after the transfusion.

Hazardous Waste Disposal

Blood centers are accustomed to dealing with biohazardous waste, but many outpatient facilities and physicians' offices are not. Because the blood components originated with the blood center, it is the center's responsibility to ascertain the final disposition of the blood and all potentially blood-contaminated materials. Blood centers deal with this issue in various ways. Greatest control is possible if the center requires the outside facility to return all contaminated materials to the blood center for disposal. The blood center then incurs the cost (which may not be easily recoverable). Another option is to obtain a copy of the agency's policy for disposal of such waste and of the contract with an approved biohazardous waste company or hospital that agrees to handle the waste. When the transfusion is performed in the home, it is particularly important to emphasize the need to leave no area contaminated and to dispose of nothing in the household garbage. Even uncontaminated items, if known to be associated with a blood transfusion, will cause concern if discovered later by nonmedical personnel.

Summary

Traditional assumptions about how care should be delivered are being reevaluated in all areas of medicine. Transfusion should be no exception. There are acceptable mechanisms to make such services available that do not require hospitalization for a specified patient population. In view of the greater risk of performing any medical procedure in an outpatient setting, it is incumbent on any blood center that wishes to become involved in providing out-of-hospital transfusion services to design its system carefully, accepting only the highest standard of medical practice and requiring rigorous quality assurance. Although this may require considerable expenditure of blood center resources, particularly in the beginning, this cost should be weighed against the significant benefit it provides for many individual patients and for the nation's attempts at health-care cost containment.

References

1. Rabiner SF, Telfer MC, Fajardo R. Home transfusion for patients with hemophilia A. N Engl J Med 1970;283:1011-15.

2. Snyder EL, Menitove JE, eds. Home transfusion therapy. Arlington, VA: American Association of Blood Banks, 1986:xi-xii.
3. Weinberg DS, Murray HW. Coping with AIDS. N Engl J Med 1987;317:1469-72.
4. Chen RT, Rutherford GW, Payne SF, et al. Use of hospitals by patients with AIDS in San Francisco. N Engl J Med 1988; 319:1671-2.
5. Koren MJ. Home care—Who cares? N Engl J Med 1986;314: 917-20.
6. Moxley JH, Roeder PC. New opportunities for out-of-hospital health services. N Engl J Med 1984;310:193-7.
7. Guilday T. Legal considerations of home blood transfusions. In: Snyder EL, Menitove JE, eds. Home transfusion therapy. Arlington, VA: American Association of Blood Banks, 1986:41-52.
8. Silberstein LE. Quality assurance for out-of-hospital transfusion programs. In: Kurtz SR, Summers SH, Kruskall MS, eds. Improving transfusion practice: The role of quality assurance. Arlington, VA: American Association of Blood Banks, 1989:53-61.
9. Rosen NR, Bates LH, Herod G. Transfusion therapy: Improved patient care and resource utilization. Transfusion 1993;33:341-7.
10. Fisher K, Gardner K, eds. Quality and home health care: Redefining the tradition. Chicago, IL: Joint Commission on Accreditation of Healthcare Organizations, 1987.
11. Beck ML, Grindon AJ. Home transfusion therapy. Transfusion 1986;26:296-8.
12. Whorton SS, McAbee B. The future role of home transfusion for the medical and surgical patient. In: Snyder EL, Menitove JE, eds. Home transfusion therapy. Arlington, VA: American Association of Blood Banks, 1986:7-14.
13. Pinkerton PH, Coovadia AS, Goldstein J. Frequency of delayed hemolytic transfusion reactions following antibody screening and immediate-spin crossmatching. Transfusion 1992;32:814-17.
14. Wentz B, Burns ER. Improvement in transfusion safety using a new blood unit and patient identification system as part of safe transfusion practice. Transfusion 1991;31:401-3.
15. Sazama K. Reports of 355 transfusion-associated deaths: 1976 through 1985. Transfusion 1990;30:583-90.
16. The Paul Gann Blood Safety Act. California Health and Safety Code. Section 1645;1991.
17. DePalma L, Snyder EL. Medical aspects of home transfusion. In: Snyder EL, Menitove JE, eds. Home transfusion therapy.

Arlington, VA: American Association of Blood Banks, 1986: 25-40.
18. Bachert LB. Making home transfusions work. Med Lab Observer 1987;19:42-6.

Additional Reading

McCann BA, Hill KL. The JCAH Home Care Project. Qual Rev Bul 1986;12(5):91-193.

Smit Sibinga CT, Das PC, Greenwalt TJ, eds. Future developments in blood banking. Boston: Martinus Nijhoff, 1986.

In: Fridey JL, Kasprisin CA and Issitt LA, eds.
Out-of-Hospital Transfusion Therapy
Bethesda, MD: American Association of Blood Banks, 1994

3

Out-of-Hospital Transfusions: Home Transfusion Therapy Programs

Lynn Douglas, BSN, RN

DURING THE LAST DECADE, home transfusion therapy has been practiced more frequently and it has been suggested that the effectiveness and safety of home transfusions may be similar to that of the hospital or ambulatory setting. Several factors associated with home care have a positive impact on the therapeutic value and beneficial effects of a transfusion. These include:

- Conservation of patient energy
- Decreased risk of exposure to infection
- Positive psychological effect of reducing the "sick" image associated with hospitalization
- A one-on-one nurse-patient relationship

In addition, with the current health-care climate, the cost savings of home care over hospitalization cannot be ignored.

Home transfusion therapy is becoming an increasingly common practice. The fact that the outcome has, thus far, been positive could be due, in part, to the high standards and stringent protocols practiced during the pioneer years of home transfusion therapy. A joint effort by home care and blood center personnel will be required to maintain this record of safety and effectiveness as the practice expands into increasing numbers of home care agencies and blood centers.

This chapter provides an overview of the areas to be addressed by a home care company in the planning, development and implementation of a home transfusion therapy program. Specific components

Lynn Douglas, BSN, RN, General Manager, Best Care Medical, Arlington, Texas necessary for a safe and successful program are discussed. The goal of this chapter is twofold: to assist the home care agency in creating and managing a home transfusion therapy program and to provide blood centers a working model to use in selecting home care companies with which to work and in creating its protocols for the provision of blood products to be used in the home care setting.

It is essential that the home care provider, whether a nursing agency or an infusion therapy company, recognize transfusion therapy as a specialty and develop its program accordingly.

Home Health-Blood Center Relationship

A vital, and possibly the most important, component of the program is the agency's relationship with a blood bank or hospital transfusion service. Open and frequent communications as well as familiarity with the practices and protocols of each are important. Attendance at blood center educational programs by home care staff and participation of blood center personnel in the home care training programs are both excellent ways to promote this relationship. Transfusion therapy in the home care setting is provided by a team. Each participant's responsibility is vital and a team approach increases the likelihood of a safe outcome. A less therapeutic outcome, of course, reflects on both entities. Therefore, a solid relationship with open lines of communication between the home care company and the blood supplier is a must.

Policy and Procedures

Another area of crucial importance to the success of a home transfusion therapy program is the need for policies and procedures specific to transfusion therapy. These should clearly define staff requirements, patient acceptance criteria, blood product procurement and the transfusion process itself.

Clinical Staff

The knowledge base and clinical skills of the registered nurses assigned to the home transfusion therapy program can, without a doubt, "make or break" the program. Standards addressing the criteria for hiring and assigning nurses should be specific and in writing. The home care company must not compromise or renege on these standards, even if it means declining a patient referral or delaying the implementation of the program. Standards should address the qualifications of nurses assigned to the transfusion therapy program, including IV skills, blood component knowledge and clinical experience. An internal certification program that includes an initial orientation program, a preceptorship and regularly scheduled in-service training specific to transfusion therapy helps ensure properly prepared personnel and may prove to be a valuable investment from a risk management perspective. The orientation program should include instructions in the areas listed in Table 3-1.

After successfully completing the general orientation class, the nurse is then supervised through at least one complete transfusion. It is recommended that independent care be provided by the nurse only after the satisfactory completion of this process.

Attendance by the nurse at the ongoing in-service training programs should be a requirement for continued assignment to transfusion therapy patients.

Patient Acceptance Criteria

In addition to the home care company's general acceptance criteria for home care, there must be a specific written policy addressing patient appropriateness for home transfusion therapy.

The patient's physician or designee must be available by telephone during the time of the transfusion. A responsible adult should be present during and for 24 hours following the transfusion. To facilitate the transfusion, the patient's home should have ample space, as well as light and electricity. A working telephone and proximity to emergency medical services (EMS) are essential.

Table 3-1. Nursing Orientation to Home Transfusion Therapy

- All company protocols, policies and procedures
- Basic blood physiology/hematology
- Patient selection
- Patient assessment
- Type and crossmatch procedure
- Procurement and transportation of blood components
- Patient and donor unit identification
- Administration protocol
- Patient monitoring
- Adverse reactions, recognition and interventions
- Patient education

The patient acceptance policy may also address the maximum number of units the patient requires. It is generally agreed upon that a patient is not acceptable for home care if his/her need exceeds three units of red blood cells (RBCs). A greater need suggests that the patient may not be stable enough for home transfusion, and also affects the time required to accomplish the complete therapy, which may diminish its cost-effectiveness. The home care company may or may not choose to limit the maximum platelet requirement.

As discussed in previous chapters, the transfusion must be clinically indicated. The patient's hemoglobin, hematocrit and/or platelet level should be appropriate for the transfusion ordered, based upon laboratory results obtained within the previous 5-7 days.

There must be adequate venous access and the patient's diagnosis should be appropriate for management in the home setting. Obviously, for example, acute blood loss is not an appropriate indication for home care. However, anemia secondary to such chronic diseases as renal failure, AIDS or bone marrow failure, or to chemotherapy can generally be treated in the home.

Physician Orders

A specific home transfusion therapy policy should define exactly what information is necessary from the patient's managing physician before blood products can be given in the home. In addition to orders for therapy, the physician should provide the patient's latest laboratory results. Orders must include the blood component to be administered, the number of units, the date to be given and the venous access route. If pretransfusion medications are indicated, the physician orders should include the drug, dose and route. Another safety precaution is to require that the physician give specific orders before the transfusion for management of a transfusion reaction. The home care company may write its policy to include the requirement that the physician inform the home care company of where he/she can be reached during the time of the transfusion. The policy should also state whether verbal orders may be followed or whether written and signed orders must be obtained before the transfusion.

Patient and Donor Compatibility and Identification

The home care company must have a very clear policy and a written step-by-step protocol that reflect the standard of care and regulations applicable to the area and that are congruent with the policies and procedures of the blood source. This policy must be followed without exception. A system for patient identification must be defined in this policy. The wristband system is the most common and probably the safest system.

It is imperative that there be rigid standards in place for the identification of the blood specimen drawn for type and crossmatch. Again, this protocol should follow the protocol of the blood center supplying the blood.

Written policy should also define the procedure for identification of the blood component at the time it is received from blood center personnel, as well as for rechecking the unit identification with the patient identification once in the patient's home.

Transport

Procedures for transporting both the specimen drawn for type and crossmatch as well as the blood component itself should comply with all federal, state and local regulations pertinent to the transport of biohazardous materials. Also, a policy should address the safe storage and transport of the blood component with specific reference to stability, temperature of the transport container and time parameters. This policy must be congruent with that of the blood source.

Patient Assessment

It is recommended that each patient be assessed specifically for home transfusion therapy within 24 hours before the scheduled transfusion. The purposes of this assessment are to determine if the patient meets acceptance criteria and to provide clinical information necessary for the safe administration of blood products. The assessment should, ideally, be performed by the nurse who will administer the actual transfusion. The completed assessment form should be in the patient's home at the time of the transfusion.

Information that is important to obtain during a pretransfusion assessment includes: name of adult caregiver; local emergency facility; physician's name and phone number; current clinical information such as medications, diagnosis, laboratory values, vital signs, mental status and cardiorespiratory stability; previous transfusion history; and venous access.

Patient Education

Specific policies regarding the education of the patient and the patient's family or significant adult are necessary. Such policies should require not only that extensive verbal instruction be given before the transfusion, but also that written materials be left with the patient. This material should be easy to read and understand, and include information about side effects and complications that may occur and what is to be done in the event of their occurrence. Written patient educational materials should always include telephone numbers for EMS as well as for the home care company. (Examples of patient educational materials are provided at the end of this chapter.)

The policy governing education of the patient might also include a procedure for receiving the patient's acknowledgment that the instruction occurred and that the patient understood. Requirements for consent for home care and for consent for blood transfusions vary from state to state. The company policy should comply with the state requirements and practices within the community.

Transfusion Administration

A written clinical procedure must be in place that specifically outlines the process for the actual blood component transfusion. This policy should specify company directives on the use of filters, the use of an infusion pump or rate control device, parameters for the rate of infusion, other fluids to be used, inspection of product, etc. The procedure also outlines patient monitoring protocols. It is important to consider that emergency assistance may be less accessible in the home care setting and that the earliest possible recognition of complications reduces the risk and severity of an adverse reaction. It is recommended that vital signs be taken just before the initiation of the transfusion, every 10 minutes for the first 30 minutes of the transfusion, and every 30 minutes thereafter. This should be repeated with the start of each separate unit. The infusion site should be observed regularly as should the overall status of the patient. Lung auscultation should be performed each time that vital signs are taken.

Posttransfusion procedures and follow-up care can be covered in this policy, and include patient instructions, reassessment procedures, and biohazardous waste transport and disposal. The posttransfusion assessment may be conducted by telephone the following day or, depending upon the status of the patient, may require another home visit. The documentation standards, expectations and protocols should be defined in this policy.

Reaction Protocol

The policy outlining actions to be taken in the event of an adverse reaction to the transfusion should include the receiving physician's orders before the transfusion, nursing interventions, administration of medications, initiation of cardiopulmonary resuscitation and contacting EMS, and documentation procedures. The home health company may institute a single policy with generic guidelines, or may have a group of clinical procedures, each covering a separate type of reaction.

Documentation

A third area of importance is documentation. It is recommended that, rather than attempting to adapt generic home care documents, transfusion-specific forms should be utilized in a home transfusion therapy program. The use of transfusion-specific forms adds a level of safety and quality to the program by alerting and sensitizing the practitioners involved in the process, from the ordering physician to the hands-on nurse.

Transfusion-specific medical record documents may include: physician's orders, nursing assessment, patient consent, transfusion record, reaction report and patient educational material.

Quality Assessment and Continuous Improvement

Finally, a successful home transfusion therapy program will have a quality assessment and continuous improvement (QACI) program. This may be a separate program specific to transfusions, or may be incorporated into the overall QA program of the home health company. Either way, there should be transfusion-specific outcome monitors, including: compliance with patient acceptance criteria, frequency and type of complications and effectiveness.

The procedure for the QACI program varies from agency to agency. An audit of 100% of the transfusions administered is suggested for all transfusion programs, especially those that are new or relatively small. The program may include a concurrent or retrospective review.

Participation and involvement of blood center personnel in the home health agency or infusion therapy company's QACI program can be helpful. Such participation could be in the form of a quarterly meeting to review outcome and recommend corrective actions or, at least, a regularly scheduled summary report to the blood center.

Financial Considerations

Before implementation of a home transfusion program, a thorough investigation of cost and reimbursement is warranted. Due to its time intensity, home transfusion therapy may be a "break even" endeavor. For example, the pretransfusion visit, type and crossmatch, obtaining the blood component, travel, the transfusion visit, documentation and follow-up care may involve 8-12 hours of skilled nursing time. The cost of the blood product, supplies and equipment must then be added to the cost of nursing hours.

Reimbursement for home transfusions varies widely among third party payers, depending on specific policy benefit structure, company philosophy and the level of managed care. In this era of cost-containment and heavily managed care, reimbursement for transfusions in the home setting seldom provides significant profit margins. Third party payers often reimburse a package rate that does not adequately cover all expenses. For example, in some areas of the country an average reimbursement may be as little as $400, while 10 hours of nursing care in the home may cost $200 and the blood product another $200.

Medicaid reimbursement varies from state to state and should be investigated on a local level. Medicare does not currently reimburse for home transfusion therapy.

Despite what may be a negative direct financial impact, infusion therapy companies are often willing to provide home transfusions for several reasons. It is perceived that the ability to perform this high-tech therapy positions the company as a leader in the industry. Also, home transfusion therapy capability gives the company a more complete product line and may encourage referral of more profitable therapies.

To maintain a desirable cost to reimbursement ratio, it is important to verify insurance benefits and obtain pricing approval before the transfusion, to manage time and supplies carefully, and to secure cost-effective product procurement.

Summary

The ideal home transfusion process involves an entire team of professionals. There are many approaches to establishing a home transfusion therapy program. This chapter offers recommendations and information that should be helpful in attaining the common goal for all home transfusion therapy programs: SAFE AND THERAPEUTIC OUTCOMES.

Acknowledgments

The author would like to thank the following individuals for their assistance in the preparation of this chapter: Alice Illian, MSN, RN, Coordinator of Staff Development and Education, CURAFLEX Health Services, Houston, TX; Ellen O'Daniel, MT(ASCP), Director of Technical Services, Carter Blood Bank, Ft. Worth, TX; Margie Peschel, MD, Medical Director, Carter Blood Bank, Ft. Worth, TX; and Kathleen Crocker, MSN, RN, CNSN, Vice President, Clinical Operations, Critical Care America, Westchester, MA.

Suggested Reading

Crocker K, Coker MH. Initiation of a home hemotherapy program using a primary nursing model. Intraven Nurs 1991;13:13-19.

Intravenous nursing standards of practice. Belmont, MA: Intravenous Nurses' Society, 1990.

Marek K, McVan B. Home transfusion therapy, an alternative. Cambridge: National Intravenous Therapy Association, 1986.

Monks N. Home transfusion therapy. J Intraven Nur, 1989;11:389-96.

Silberstein L, ed. Out-of-hospital transfusions. Arlington, VA: American Association of Blood Banks, 1989.

Appendix 3-1. Home Transfusion Therapy Visit Report—Clinical Note

HOME TRANSFUSION THERAPY
VISIT REPORT - CLINICAL NOTE

PATIENT NAME ______________________ ID#______________ DATE__________

BLOOD TYPE: ABO__________ Rh_____ hgb ______ hct ______ date _____

PHYSICIAN'S NAME______________________________

VENOUS ACCESS TYPE ____________________ DATE INSERTED__________

SITE ASSESSMENT____

IV SOLUTION______________________ TIME BEGUN________

PREMEDICATIONS:	medication	dose	route	time
	____________	________	______	______
	____________	________	______	______

BLOOD COMPONENT:	unit ID #	type	time start/stop	volume
	____________	______	__________	______
	____________	______	__________	______
	____________	______	__________	______

NOTES:	time	BP	T	P	R	lungs	comment
	____	____	___	___	___	________	______________
	____	____	___	___	___	________	______________
	____	____	___	___	___	________	______________
	____	____	___	___	___	________	______________
	____	____	___	___	___	________	______________
	____	____	___	___	___	________	______________
	____	____	___	___	___	________	______________
	____	____	___	___	___	________	______________
	____	____	___	___	___	________	______________
	____	____	___	___	___	________	______________
	____	____	___	___	___	________	______________
	____	____	___	___	___	________	______________

PATIENT RESPONSE ____
____
____
____

PATIENT INSTRUCTIONS ____
____

PLAN ____
____

signature____ date______

Appendix 3-2. Home Transfusion Assessment

HOME TRANSFUSION ASSESSMENT

DATE ________

NAME ____________________ ACCT # ________ DOB ________

ADDRESS ______________________________ PHONE ________

CAREGIVER AVAILABLE ______________ RELATIONSHIP ________

EMS # __________ EMERGENCY FACILITY ______________

PHYSICIAN ____________________ PHONE ________

DATE LAST SEEN __________

PRIMARY DIAGNOSIS ______________ DATE OF ONSET ________

REASON FOR TRANSFUSION ______________________

OTHER DIAGNOSIS __________________________

CURRENT MEDICATIONS ________________________

____

ALLERGIES ______________________________

HGB _____ HCT _____ PLATELETS ________ DATE DRAWN ________

BP ______ T ______ mental status ________

P ______ R ______ ________________

cardio-resp __________ other ______________

__________ ______________

__________ ______________

PREVIOUS TRANSFUSION ____Y ____N DATE OF LAST ________

BLOOD PRODUCT TRANSFUSED ________________

TRANSFUSION REACTION ___Y ___N explain ______________

____

BLOOD TYPE: ABO ________ Rh ______

VENOUS ACCESS ______________________________

____

T & CM DRAWN ____________________

PATIENT/CAREGIVER INSTRUCTIONS ___Y ___N CONSENT ___Y ___N

ACCEPTABLE FOR HOME TRANSFUSION ___Y ___N

COMMENT ______________________________

DATE TO BE TRANSFUSED __________ # UNITS ________

BLOOD COMPONENTS ______________________

SIGNATURE ______________________ DATE ________

Appendix 3-3. Home Transfusion Physician's Orders

HOME TRANSFUSION

PHYSICIAN'S ORDERS

NAME ______________________________ ACCT # __________

PREVIOUS TRANSFUSION REACTION ____Y ____N explain ______________

____

HGB ________ HCT ________ PLATELETS __________ LAB DATE __________

ORDERS:

1. Admit to Home Health services for RN to assess, prepare, instruct and administer Home Transfusion Therapy
2. Type & Cross Match __________ units RBC

   Type __________ units platelets; other ______________
3. Venous access ______________________________
4. Date to be transfused __________
5. Pre transfusion medications

   med dose route

   ____

   ____

   ____
6. Post transfusion lab ______________________________
7. Transfusion Reaction orders:

   ___PRN medications: ___Benadryl 25-50 mg po/IM prn itching, or rash

   ___Epinephrine 1:10,000 _____ml prn respiratory distress

   ___Normal Saline infusion at up to _____ml per hour prn severe hypotension

   ___Other ______________________

   ____

   ___Stop / slow transfusion

   ___Initiate EMS and follow company protocol for severe or suspected hemolytic reaction

Physician Name ______________________ Phone __________

Address ______________________________

available during transfusion ____Y ____N

Signature ______________________ date __________

Appendix 3-4. Transfusion Reaction Report

TRANSFUSION REACTION REPORT

PATIENT NAME ______________________________ACCT # _________

DATE OF TRANSFUSION __________________ TIME INITIATED _____

NUMBER UNITS ORDERED __________ NUMBER UNITS ADMINISTERED _____

PRE TRANSFUSION MEDICATIONS ___Y ___N ________________________

____

ONSET OF SYMPTOMS: TIME____ ___DURING ____AFTER UNIT # ________

SYMPTOMS:

[] FEVER
[] BACK PAIN
[] NAUSEA
[] CHILLS
[] CHEST PAIN
[] HYPOTENSION
[] ITCHING
[] WHEEZING
[] HYPERTENSION
[] HIVES/RASH
[] DYSPNEA
[] HEADACHE
[] RESTLESSNESS
[] OTHER ___________________

____

VITAL SIGNS: PRE TRANSFUSION BP _____ T _____ P _____ R _____

POST TRANSFUSION BP _____ T _____ P _____ R _____

ACTION TAKEN:

[] TRANSFUSION STOPPED
[] RECHECKED ID & BLOOD ID
[] NORMAL SALINE INFUSION
[] NOTIFIED BLOOD BANK

RATE __________

[] MEDICATIONS ADMINISTERED

____

____

____

[] NOTIFIED PHYSICIAN

RESPONSE: _______________

____

[] EMS ACTIVATED
[] CPR
[]OTHER

____

____

____

SENT TO LAB: [] REMAINDER OF UNIT IN QUESTION

[] REMAINING BLOOD COMPONENT UNITS

[] BLOOD SPECIMEN
[] URINE SPECIMEN

[] REACTION REPORT
[] TRANSFUSION REPORT

SIGNATURE _________________________________

Appendix 3-5. Patient Instructions—Post Blood Transfusion

PATIENT INSTRUCTIONS
POST BLOOD TRANSFUSION

Although complications following a Blood Transfusion are rare, there are some signs or symptoms of these complications that you should know. During the next 24 hours, you should rest, drink plenty of fluids if you are able, and pay particular attention to any symptoms which you had not already been experiencing.

Please call your home care RN and / or your physician if you experience any of the following symptoms:

_fever greater than 100.6 F
you should take your temperature every 4 hours during the next 24 hours

_itching, rash or hives

_pain in your chest, flank or back that you did not have before the Transfusion

_irregular heart beat

_red or dark urine

_fatigue, loss of appetite, nausea, or vomiting

_shortness of breath or difficulty breathing
IF SEVERE, CALL 911

NAMES AND TELEPHONE NUMBERS

home care RN_________________ phone ________

Physician _____________________ phone ________

EMERGENCY 911

Appendix 3-6. Patient Information—Receiving Transfusion Therapy at Home

PATIENT INFORMATION
RECEIVING TRANSFUSION THERAPY AT HOME

__ A Blood Transfusion is the introduction of blood or a blood component into the circulatory system through your vein. It can replace lost blood, increase the oxygen carrying capacity of the blood, and/or correct bleeding disorders.

__ Prior to your Transfusion a Registered Nurse with special training will visit you to explain what type of Transfusion your doctor has ordered. The nurse will ask you about your health history, will assess your current condition, and will ask you to sign a consent form for Blood Transfusion.

__ Unless you already have an Intravenous Catheter, your nurse will insert a small plastic tube (IV catheter) into your vein.

__ The nurse will also draw a sample of your blood and take it to the blood bank. To Insure transfusion of blood matched specifically with your blood, the nurse will give you a special identification wristband to wear. DO NOT REMOVE THIS WRISTBAND.

__ Prior to your Transfusion, the blood bank will determine your blood type and compare it to the donor's blood type to Insure that they are matched appropriately.

__On the day of your Transfusion, the nurse will bring the blood to your home in an insulated container and will bring all of the supplies and equipment necessary for a safe Transfusion.

__The blood will be transfused through the IV catheter inserted by your nurse, or through your ____________________. A saline solution will be started before the blood is transfused.

__The nurse will remain with you throughout the procedure, and for at least 30 minutes afterwards, measuring your temperature, blood pressure, heart rate and respirations frequently.

__ At the end of the Transfusion, the nurse will fully instruct you and a family member about possible complications and what you should do during the 24 hours following the Transfusion.

__Most Transfusions are tolerated quite well. However, reactions can occur. These range from very mild itching, flushing of the face, fever and chills to chest pain and shortness of breath. Your nurse has been trained and has your doctor's approval to treat these symptoms appropriately.

In: Fridey JL, Kasprisin CA and Issitt LA, eds.
Out-of-Hospital Transfusion Therapy
Bethesda, MD: American Association of Blood Banks, 1994

4

Out-of-Hospital Transfusion: Financial Perspectives

Virginia Vengelen-Tyler, MBA, MT(ASCP)SBB

OUT-OF-HOSPITAL TRANSFUSION (OHT) of blood and blood components has become more common as a result of recent advancements in outpatient treatments and a desire to provide better patient service. In the 1980's, hospitals needed to deliver appropriate quality medical care within the boundaries of imposed fiscal restraints. Government-established limits determined reimbursement based on diagnosis-related groups (DRGs). Similarly, insurance companies established reimbursement limits based on their monthly or annual payments. Health maintenance organizations (HMOs) also established reimbursement limits based on annual premiums paid by members. These reforms resulted in a need to reduce hospital stays for patients, while providing safe and cost-effective alternatives. Outpatient clinics added transfusion services to their venue, and out-of-hospital health-care services added transfusions to their list of therapies.

The development of programs using alternative locations for transfusing patients must take several measurements into account. First, the health-care provider must be able to provide the same safe and quality service at about the same, or preferably lower, cost than is available in the hospital. The payer must accept the new policies, and may expect to pay less for the service. Finally, society should benefit as a whole by the delivery of safe health care at either a reduced or acceptable cost for the services provided.

Providers offering OHT services will need to evaluate several aspects of the costs and benefits OHT services will provide for the

Virginia Vengelen-Tyler, MBA, MT(ASCP)SBB, Laboratory Services Manager, San Diego Blood Bank, San Diego, California patient. The decision to start an OHT program should be based on a clear understanding of the medical procedures, ancillary treatments, space requirements, as well as insurance, legal and start-up costs. These costs should be balanced against the benefits of the program, or that part of the program in which a "contracting agency" participates.

The information presented in this chapter explores areas to consider when developing a business plan for analyzing an existing service or creating a new service. Suggestions on how to perform financial analysis for an OHT program and possible strategies for future OHT services are also presented.

Needs Assessment

Needs of the Community

Before any plans are made to provide a service, there must be a need in the community for that service. The most compelling need for an OHT program is to provide a safe and less expensive method of care for a well-defined patient population. For instance, OHT programs provide a great service to the elderly and patients suffering from AIDS-related illnesses, by providing blood transfusion in the familiar home environment. Many patients already benefiting from home health care are terminally or chronically ill, and prefer treatment at home or with family in attendance at a local clinic.[1-4] Offering transfusions at home may not extend the lives of patients, but it can improve the quality of their lives by not requiring travel or ambulance transport to hospitals in order to receive scheduled transfusions. OHT programs also provide a more humane treatment of the elderly, patients with AIDS and others. The option of being transfused out-of-hospital may reduce such stresses as being wheeled through a hospital setting or sitting in waiting rooms for treatment.

Others who benefit from OHT programs are chronically transfused patients such as those suffering from thalassemia, sickle cell disease, chronic anemia and leukemia. The OHT program provides one-on-one contact with the health-care giver and the patient, thus possibly providing a personal service greater than that available in the hospital.

The difference in cost between out-of-hospital and in-hospital transfusions is very difficult to assess, in part because it is hard to place a monetary value on improving the *quality* of a patient's life. For some patients, it could include calculation of labor costs involved in time lost from the patient's place of employment, or it might mean the difference between illness-related unemployment or ability to keep a job. Most of these potential benefits to the patient do not have an easily calculated dollar value.

Needs of the Physician

In addition to there being a need in the community for an OHT program, physicians must also acknowledge a need for such a program. The physician must balance various aspects of patient care relative to the safety of the procedures. The physician may be receptive to ordering the service if the patient's well-being and diagnosis supports use of OHT. If OHT provides a needed service to the patient, at no increase in cost or inconvenience to the patient, and will be covered by the patient's insurance in a manner similar to in-hospital coverage, then the physician may consider ordering the service.

Some physicians offer transfusion services in their offices or clinics. In these cases, all claims for Medicare and Medicaid are handled through the physician's office. Crossmatching and providing blood and blood products are contracted to hospitals or blood centers. In some cases, infusion nursing services are also contracted by the physician's office to transfuse the patients in the office. Whichever method of transfusion is used, when transfusions are given in a physician's office, that office should utilize trained IV phlebotomists or transfusionists to administer the transfusions, and emergency facilities should be available if needed. Offering transfusions in this setting may reduce costs to the patient.

Needs of the Facility Supplying the Service

Any facility providing OHT services or any portion of that service must be able to meet the needs of the contracting agency without increasing net expenses to the transfusion facility. In other words, such activities must break even or increase revenues.

All health-care services must be cost efficient. In some cases, providing a transfusion service may be part of an overall package of services. Offering a transfusion service may allow for greater opportunities to increase a facility's patient base or the volume of cost-effective services. For example, a home health care agency may offer OHT to patients previously denied the services at home. Also, OHT may provide another needed therapy (blood transfusion) to cancer patients already receiving chemotherapy at home. The transfusion service offered by these agencies, even when offered as part of a package, must not cost more than it collects in revenues.

Projected Program Costs

What are some of the costs to consider before developing an OHT service? A partial list of direct and indirect costs is outlined in Table 4-1. Costs are divided into three groups: those for hospital-based transfusion services, those for blood-center-based transfusion services and those for home health care agencies. Although there are several similarities among these services, there are also some differences in costs required to run the programs and in amounts of reimbursement. Currently, outpatient and in-home transfusions are being offered or contracted out by all three of the groups listed.

Hospital-Based Transfusion Services

The hospital-based transfusion service can offer a variety of transfusion options. It can offer transfusion services to hospital outpatient clinics, other hospitals, clinics or home health care agencies.

Hospital-based outpatient centers can reduce the costs of transfusion services below those that would be incurred if patients were admitted to a hospital for their chronic transfusion needs.[2-3] These centers are usually housed in, or close to, the hospital and usually fall under the management of the hospital administration. This arrangement may help reduce overhead costs of the service as these costs are shared by multiple hospital cost centers.

Most of the costs for a hospital transfusion service providing OHT to an outpatient area are outlined in Table 4-1. The costs for packaging and delivery of the blood to the outpatient setting may not apply if the outpatient facility is in the same building as the transfusion service. Some costs in the outpatient service, such as those for occupying space, are determined by formulas set by the hospital. A typical formula is:

$$\frac{\text{Total rental (cost center)}}{\text{\% of time used for OHT}} = \text{rental cost for OHT}$$

Table 4-1. Comparative Costs for Out-of-Hospital Transfusion Services

	Hospital Transfusion Service	Blood Center	Home Health Care Agency
DIRECT COSTS:			
Fixed Costs:			
Nursing Services: Administrative staff Medical staff Billing staff Compliance/QA staff	Yes	Yes	Yes
Laboratory Service: Administrative staff Medical staff Billing staff Compliance/QA staff	Yes	Yes	Contract
Variable Costs:			
Nursing Services: Nursing labor costs Supplies/filters/administration sets Paperwork	Yes	Yes	Yes
Laboratory Services: Technologist labor costs Reagents, supplies Paperwork	Yes	Yes	Contract
Delivery Service: Taxi, or "for hire" transportation service Existing service employed at facility	If shipped	If shipped	Yes
Packaging: Labor Ice or coolant QC of containers for shipping blood	If shipped	If shipped	NA
INDIRECT COSTS:			
Building rental (portion of facilities cost)	Yes	Yes	Yes
Insurance	Yes	Yes	Yes
Equipment depreciation	Yes	Yes	Yes
Preventive maintenance contracts on equipment (etc)	Yes	Yes	Yes
Legal services (liability for facility and for performing services of OHT)	Yes	Yes	Yes

Similar formulas exist for other indirect costs. Insurance and legal costs should be allocated appropriately to the OHT cost center. If exclusive insurance and legal expenses are incurred for the OHT program, they should be added to the OHT cost center. The cost of emergency equipment acquired for this service must also be added to the OHT cost center. If these services or costs are shared with other activities or cost centers, then they must be divided among the cost centers in an equitable manner.

A hospital-based transfusion service can also act as a contract service for a health-care provider not affiliated with the hospital. Providing OHT in this manner can be a financially safe service because the costs incurred by the hospital are predetermined, based on calculated expenses. These costs are billed directly to the health-care provider without costly and time-consuming completion of reimbursement forms. The primary costs incurred by offering this service would be the direct and indirect costs of the laboratory performing the service. Once these costs are calculated, it is a simple matter of billing the health-care provider. Some indirect costs to keep in mind are additional insurance and legal costs that may be incurred by the hospital in providing the transfusion service. These costs must be added as indirect costs. In some hospitals, this service is offered only when the ordering physician is on staff at the hospital. In these cases, the need for the hospital to carry additional insurance may not be necessary.

An additional cost that hospital transfusion services must consider is the expense of packaging and shipping the blood. As the supplier of the blood or blood products, the hospital must provide a safe and controlled environment for the transport of the blood. It is the responsibility of the transfusion service to ensure that the agency's quality control records are appropriate when the agency provides the shipping containers. These records must document proper shipping and storage temperature for the products.

Many HMOs and community hospitals provide full outpatient or in-home transfusion services to staff physicians' patients.[2] A cost center should be developed to identify and compile the costs of these services. The OHT service can be made into a separate cost center or department, and services required for this cost center can be subcontracted within the hospital. For example, laboratory costs could account for 15% of the costs, pharmacy 12%, nursing 60%, billing 8%, etc. The ultimate objectives of these services are to provide a complete patient care package and to offer "full service patient care" for the physicians. The costs involved in this type of service are the same as those outlined for home health care agencies in Table 4-1. Specialized costs for this service are discussed late in the home health agency section.

Blood-Center-Based Transfusion Services

OHT services provided by blood centers have helped physicians care for anemic patients at home and provided a service generally unavailable elsewhere. Until the present, many blood centers had not established programs for transfusing patients on an outpatient basis in their own blood center. This was due to the fact that blood centers were not equipped or staffed to provide the individual care needed for transfusions. In some instances, this service was provided because of state licensure requirements or reimbursement limits. As insurance agencies and state governments review alternative methods for health care, some of these obstacles are being removed. Some blood centers are now positioning themselves to provide these services to the entire community. The projected costs for blood centers are listed in Table 4-1.

The development of alternative locations for transfusions has provided new opportunities for blood centers to enter the patient services arena. Some blood centers have developed out-of-hospital services similar to those provided by a hospital and are beginning to include both outpatient transfusions and in-home care. The recent increase in demand to collect autologous blood from patients who would not qualify as normal healthy blood donors and the associated necessary medical oversight have helped blood centers prepare for this change in philosophy.

A blood center embarking on the development of an outpatient care facility must be committed to patient care and perceive a need in the community for these services. Blood centers are in a unique position because they may fulfill a community need by providing OHT services to a larger geographic area than most hospitals can offer. Also, blood centers may be able to provide these services for physicians on staff at hospitals not providing OHT services.

Costs involved in developing these services vary depending upon the individual programs. Overhead costs may be shared with the blood center, or a separate facility that would use some of the blood center's services could be developed. These costs would be similar to those of a transfusion service providing outpatient care and a home health care agency providing in-home transfusions. (See Table 4-1.)

Blood centers can also offer laboratory testing and crossmatching for home health care agencies. Many blood centers provide this service to a large number of home health care agencies over a wide geographic area. One cost that might be lower for blood centers than hospital-based transfusion services is the cost of packaging and shipping the blood. These costs are spread over a larger number of blood products and may be fairly low. Costs to consider for this service would be the laboratory direct and indirect costs as outlined in Table 4-1.

Home Health Care Agency

Home health care agencies provide a number of services to patients at home, such as intravenous therapy, chemotherapy, care of AIDS patients and special care of terminally ill patients. Their established expertise in intravenous therapy and treatment of chronically anemic patients formed a basis for adding blood transfusions to the services already provided by these agencies. However, an OHT service, including pre- and posttransfusion visits, is much more labor-intensive than most other services offered by visiting nurses. For this reason, transfusions are usually offered as a package service to patients requiring other in-home treatments. Some of the costs incurred by this group are outlined in Table 4-1.

Several costs unique to home health care agencies are those involved in pre- and posttransfusion blood sample collection (see Table 4-2). A nurse must make a special trip to the patient's home to collect the pretransfusion blood samples. The costs of these trips include travel time, mileage, time at the patient's home, time needed to complete paperwork (including consent for transfusion) and preparations for the transfusion the following day. This generates considerable labor costs and is billed under incurred transfusion expenses. Unless other treatments can be combined with these visits, costs for transfusion alone can become very high. Additional costs on the day of the transfusion include the nurse's travel time, set-up time for the transfusion and the time required to prepare for an emergency, such as making sure a physician is available by phone. Once the transfusion is started, the nurse provides one-on-one care during the entire transfusion. Finally, the nurse's time is required for collecting posttransfusion blood samples, if needed, and patient evaluation. Again, these expenses are billed as nursing time.

The laboratory services required by home health care agencies are obtained by contracting with outside laboratories or

Table 4-2. Comparative, Direct Costs for Pre- and Posttransfusion Blood Sample Collection and Transfusion

	Home Care Agency	Hospital or Blood Center
Nursing travel time to collect the pretransfusion sample and administer the transfusion	Yes	No
Additional set-up time to ensure all emergency care resources are available	Yes	No
Actual transfusion time (one-on-one care)	Yes	Maybe
One-hour posttransfusion surveillance for reactions	Yes	Maybe
Posttransfusion visit to draw blood and evaluate patient	Yes	No

transfusion services. These costs are usually billed directly to the home health care agency. Additional indirect costs could be incurred by these agencies if they need to increase their existing insurance coverage in order to provide transfusion services. Also, additional legal services may be required to contract with hospitals or blood centers for their participation.

Investment Analysis

Break-Even Analysis

In order for any facility to offer a service, it must be proven that revenues will offset expenses. In some instances, the new service may be given an initial start-up period with increased outlay of funds but eventually (usually within 2-3 years) that service must begin to break even financially or show a profit.

> *The break-even point is a measure of the quantity of procedures needed to generate enough revenue to cover all fixed and variable costs.*

Within this calculation, several factors must be considered. Which expenses are attributable to the given services? Which expenses remain fixed and which expenses vary based on the number of services performed? At a given volume, additional staff may need to be hired. If the new staff member is dedicated to the department, then salary and benefits may be considered fixed. If the staff member is only going to be used on an as-needed basis, then his or her salary and benefits would be a variable cost. Judgments need to be made on these and other such expenses. Simply expressed, the break-even point would be calculated as shown by the example in Fig 4-1.

In order for an OHT service to operate efficiently and economically, that service must offer OHT at a fair cost. Those costs are determined by calculating the expenses incurred in providing these services, as outlined earlier in this chapter. These expenses must be passed on to the patient or payer. Alternative means for supporting a program, such as outside grants, may be considered. In most organizations, if a service is to break even, there must be enough volume to make it worthwhile to provide that service. When the volume of OHT drops below the break-even level for any period of

Out-of-Hospital Service

Variable Cost (per procedure)	
Salary	$50.00
Benefits	15.00
Supplies	30.00
Total variable cost	$95.00
Fixed Cost (monthly)	
Lease expense	$500.00
Telephone	40.00
Utilities	70.00
Depreciation expense	200.00
Total fixed cost	$810.00

Fee per procedure $120.00

Break-even volume for the out-of-hospital service charged at $120 is:

$120 (Y) = $810 + $95 (Y)

Y = 32.4 procedures per month

Figure 4-1. Calculation of the break-even point. The fee per procedure × volume (Y) = fixed costs + [variable cost × volume (Y)].

time, the facility's management will need to assess if it should continue to offer this service. The break-even analysis provides management with the volume of OHT required to make the program cost-efficient. As a result of performing the break-even analysis, management may decide that the program is necessary, but that improvement in services is needed in order to compete with organizations offering the same service. In this case, additional expenses may need to be incurred in order to achieve the goal of added volume. Appropriate marketing strategies may help facilities determine if these additional expenditures would improve the financial outlook, and what the real need for these services is in the community.

Return on Investment

Another measurement of financial well-being is the return on investment (ROI). The ROI is one of the most important ratios used when evaluating a service because it incorporates the two fundamental factors that are inherent in measuring profitability: earnings and investment. A good or healthy ROI is achieved when income will pay for the investment within a set period of time. The ROI is computed by dividing income by the amount of investment. A sample ROI calculation is shown in Fig 4-2.

Revenue (50 procedures @ $120)		$6,000.00
Expenses:		
Variable (50 procedures @ $95)	4,750.00	
Fixed	810.00	
Total expenses	5,560.00	
Monthly income (revenue less expenses)		$440.00
Annual income (12 months @ $440)		$5,280.00
Investment in equipment	$12,000.00	

Rate of return = Annual income /Investment in equipment

Rate of return = $5,280/$12,000 = 44%

Figure 4-2. Calculation of return on investment, using the costs from the break-even analysis in Fig 4-1 with a volume of 50 procedures per month.

The ability of a service to earn a satisfactory income and ROI is an important factor of good financial "health." In order for a facility to show good financial health, it should pay off the equipment within a reasonable amount of time (usually 2-5 years). Therefore, a 44% ROI would be very good if the equipment was to be paid off in 3 years, but it would not be good if the equipment was to be paid off in 2 years. In the example shown in Fig 4-2, if the pay-off period was 2 years, adjustments would have to be made on either end of the equation to approach a 50% ROI. This can be achieved by either increasing the annual income, by increasing the cost or the volume of the service, or decreasing the investment in equipment by spreading payments over 3 years or purchasing a less expensive piece of equipment.

These formulas can be used by any of the groups providing OHT services. Each facility will have to determine its fixed and variable costs as they relate to the OHT service. Cost centers that do not break even will need to review their services to determine if they can perform services less expensively or use equipment or resources more economically. A facility providing OHT will need to redefine its charges or attempt to increase its volume of patients when the ROI is not adequate. Other strategies such as whether to contract out some services to decrease overhead or equipment costs may also need to be considered.

Cost:Benefit Analysis

Another calculation important in deciding whether to offer a service is the cost:benefit analysis. In the health-care situation requiring blood transfusions, this type of analysis is very difficult. In order to determine the cost of the service, one must put dollar values on benefits received by the patient using the service. As mentioned earlier in the chapter, this may be more easily calculated for patients who, as a result of being treated as an outpatient, can remain productive in a job or career while obtaining medical treatment.[4-5] The patient's value to society as a taxpayer and the self-esteem in being employed are more difficult to quantitate. To put a dollar value on improving the quality of life of the terminally ill is an even more difficult task.

Consideration should be given to ensuring that the burden of payment for the patient is not increased as a result of providing OHT services, if at all possible. These services should be covered by the appropriate payer, and this author believes the payments should not be higher than those billed by performing the procedure in an inpatient setting. In the case of OHT services, insurance companies may respond positively if presented with data demonstrating that these procedures are less expensive and provide a better service to the patient.

The Future

In-home health care and outpatient services will continue to flourish in the future. Large medical centers, HMOs, blood centers and independent health care agencies will all be competing for this business. In order to compete in these markets, providers must be flexible about the demands of patients, physicians and insurance companies, and the financial restraints of their own organizations. The future treatment of patients will demand more portability, equipment and products, and better data collection for patient records. Perhaps the use of laptop computers in a patient's home, connected directly to a physician's office by modem, will become commonplace. Thus, data could be transmitted from portable bedside testing equipment by the attending nurse.

The challenge to health-care providers will be to provide quality services safely, to the advantage of the patient, physician and payer. In order to achieve this goal, a comprehensive business plan must be developed to project costs and expenses. Continued technological advances and data networking will undoubtedly allow for greater growth potential of these services.

Summary

The growth of out-of-hospital services will continue. The US Department of Health and Human Services showed that in 1992, $8.5 billion was spent on home health care.[6] However, this figure does not reflect all costs of home health care because costs for physicians, laboratory services, drugs and other related fees were not included in its calculation. The figure for home infusion therapy for 1993 is estimated at $3.6 billion.[6] Home transfusion and OHT services will certainly continue to expand in the future. It will be the responsibility of facilities providing these services to do so in a manner that allows for the provision of safe and cost-effective services.

References

1. Marek K, McVan B. Home transfusion therapy: A new dimension in home care. Quality Review Bulletin 1987;1:17-20.
2. Grizzard MB, Harris G, Karns H. Use of outpatient parenteral antibiotic therapy in a health maintenance organization. Rev Infect Dis 1991;13(suppl 2):S174-9.
3. Vance JC. Day-transfusion centre for patients with thalassaemia major. Lancet 1975;1(7913):967-8.
4. Jones P. Haemophilia home therapy. Haemostasis 1992;22:247-50.
5. Han AM, Han KE, Myint TT. Thalassemia in the outpatient department of the Yangon Children's Hospital in Myanmar: Cost analysis of the day-care-room services for thalassemia. S E Asian J Trop Med Public Health 1992;23:273-7.
6. Milkovich G. Costs and benefits. Hosp Pract [Off Ed] 1993;28(suppl 1):39-43.

In: Fridey JL, Kasprisin CA and Issitt LA, eds.
Out-of-Hospital Transfusion Therapy
Bethesda, MD: American Association of Blood Banks, 1994

5

Legal Considerations for Out-of-Hospital Transfusions

Kathleen Sazama, MD, JD

PATIENT CARE IS AVAILABLE in a variety of settings, increasingly at sites away from hospitals. While these alternative settings permit increased choice for patients, providers should be mindful of any legal consequences for supporting transfusions in such settings.

Preparation

To minimize legal liability for providing out-of-hospital transfusions, it is helpful to understand the bases for lawsuits. The most common legal actions include claims of battery, negligence and/or breach of contract.

Battery

Battery is the legal basis for suing whenever one person has "touched" another without that person's consent. Note that it is not necessary for the touch to be violent or delivered with force, only that the person being touched finds it objectionable. The insertion of a needle into a patient's arm is considered battery if the patient refused or did not agree to its placement. For the out-of-hospital transfusion, the patient may claim that she/he did not agree to having the blood sample taken for crossmatch or to placement of

Kathleen Sazama, MD, JD, Professor of Pathology and Laboratory Medicine and Director of Clinical Laboratories, Medical College of Pennsylvania, Philadelphia, Pennsylvania the intravenous line for the actual transfusion, or both. Because the heart of such a lawsuit is often whether the patient agreed or consented to insertion of the needle, it has similarities to negligence actions in which lack of informed consent is claimed.

Contracts

Contracts are legally enforceable agreements between competent parties in which, for a specified consideration, there is an exchange of promises to do (or refrain to do) something. When contracts are broken, there generally is a mechanism by which the breaching party is required to compensate the party who lived up to the agreement. In medical situations, this rarely forms a basis for legal action between the patient and physician.

However, in out-of-hospital transfusion situations, contracts often define the relationship between the organization responsible for administering the transfusion and the facility supplying the appropriate blood component. These contractual relationships should clearly delineate responsibilities for harm to the patient that may arise, whether unavoidable or otherwise. The blood-supplying facility ("supplier") may be better informed than the transfusing organization ("transfuser") about both legal and regulatory requirements for transfusions, which the supplier should provide to the transfuser to ensure compliance. Because harm can arise from improper transfusion practices as early as the time of blood sample collection for crossmatching to long after the actual transfusion (for transfusion-transmitted viral diseases), responsibility for proper practices should be understood by and agreeable to both parties. The contract provides a vehicle for documenting the parties' promises for the entire arrangement.

Attorneys disagree about the length and specificity of contracts. One approach is to minimize the writing, keeping it very general; the other is to provide detailed information. Either approach is acceptable and generally depends on the parties' relationships, the longevity of the agreement, existing state laws and court decisions, and other factors. The advice of individual counsel should be sought by each of the contracting parties.

Negligence

When patients sue health-care systems (including hospitals, blood centers, clinical laboratories, doctors, other professionals, etc), the usual legal basis is negligence—specifically, medical malpractice. For the suing party (the plaintiff) to succeed, he/she must prove that the sued party (the defendant) was negligent, ie, that the defendant's breach of an existing duty to the plaintiff caused injury that is compensable (Table 5-1). To establish that the defendant was negligent, experts are required to testify about the standard of care for providing the services. When the plaintiff's injury occurs during an out-of-hospital transfusion, there may be considerable divergence of expert opinion, especially with minimal[1] or no published standards.

For each of these three legal theories, the understandings between parties to a contract, or between patient and physician, should result in some written documentation. The need for such documentation is evident when disagreements and conflicts arise.

Informed Consent

The special circumstance of providing medical services, including blood transfusion, has unique requirements legally, and involves the responsibility for showing that a physician actually ordered and the patient agreed to receive the treatment or plan of therapy that was involved in his/her injury. This interaction and its documentation are characterized as obtaining proper informed consent from the patient.[2]

The two important components of informed consent are informing the patient and obtaining his/her agreement to the proposed plan of treatment based on that information.

Informing the Patient

Whose Responsibility?

The physician who has evaluated the patient and determined a course of treatment, including out-of-hospital transfusion support,

Table 5-1. Elements of Negligence

- A duty is/was owed by the defendant
- The duty was breached
- The plaintiff was injured
- The defendant's breach of duty was the cause of the plaintiff's injury
- Payment (damages) can be calculated

is responsible for conveying such information to the patient in a manner which the patient can understand and under conditions in which the patient is encouraged to resolve any confusion about or hesitancy to accept the physician's advice. It is not acceptable to transfer the responsibility for obtaining informed consent to personnel other than the treating physician.

What Information?

As long ago as 1956, California courts have required physicians to disclose to the patient "all the facts which mutually affect his rights and interests and of the [] risk, hazard and danger, if any...".[3] The court, quoting the landmark 1914 decision in *Schloendorff v Society of New York Hospital*[4] in which a person's right to make decisions affecting his/her own body ("self-determination") was legally established in the US, further stated that a "physician violates his duty to his patient and subjects himself to liability if he withholds any facts which are necessary to form the basis of an intelligent consent by the patient to the proposed treatment. Likewise, the physician may not minimize the known dangers of a procedure or operation in order to induce his patient's consent."[2]

Subsequent cases have required physicians to explain the risks of *not* receiving therapy,[5,6] introducing the requirement that the patient be offered alternatives with a discussion of risks and benefits of these as well as of the proposed treatment.

One additional requirement is that the information be material, that is, information "which the physician knows or should know would be regarded as significant by a reasonable person in the patient's position when deciding to accept or reject the recommended medical procedure."[7]

Methods of Communication

The nature and extent of the communication between patient and physician should be tailored to meet the needs of the particular patient. For transfusion practices, it is often helpful to provide written information for the patient and his/her significant others in order to supplement the verbal interchange with the physician. The settings in which communication about out-of-hospital transfusions occur should encourage frank, nonpressured dialogue about the transfusion itself and the additional risks involved in undertaking transfusion in settings outside a hospital. Alternatives should be proposed, including, eg, having the transfusion administered in a hospital, no transfusion and other options.

Language. When the patient and family or significant others have as their primary language one other than the language native to the physician, information for consent should be provided in the patient's language when possible, using the best available interpreter/translator.

Reading Level. Scientific and medical information is often provided at a reading comprehension level of a college graduate or higher. Whenever possible, the written material that explains the risks and benefits of transfusion therapy and its alternatives should be reviewed and revised by lay persons with lesser education to improve readability and comprehension by patients whose decision to accept or reject transfusion should be based upon it.

Accuracy. Each physician who orders transfusion therapy (both in- and out-of-hospital) is responsible for the accuracy of information explaining risks and benefits of this therapy to patients. The scientific literature undergoes such rapid changes that individual physicians may find it difficult to stay current without frequent interaction with a transfusion medicine specialist. Some states (eg, California) have mandated a uniform fact sheet for transfusions to be given to each patient before transfusion. This requirement may provide some benefit to the defendant physician in litigation involving consent for transfusion.

In the particular setting of out-of-hospital transfusions, a discussion of the additional risks/benefits of the setting should also occur. The patient should be informed that, when transfusions will be administered in a clinic, ambulatory care facility, nursing home, physician office, hospice or home setting, there may be a delay in obtaining emergency care and that transfusion medicine specialists may not be readily available.

Environment Conducive to Discussion

When the physician's discussion with a patient occurs in a public setting, in a situation with numerous interruptions or in the few moments before the start of treatment, most persons would agree that the patient's consent could be challenged. Consequently, transfusion treatment should be discussed, except in emergency situations, in a setting that encourages dialogue, particularly eliciting and responding to the patient's questions and concerns. Consent obtained as a result of open discussion supports an inference of the patient's decision being based on information understood by him/her.

Obtaining Consent

Documentation

Consent occurs when the activities described above have occurred to the patient's satisfaction so that he/she agrees to the proposed transfusion. Evidence of such consent is usually manifested by the patient's (or a legally qualified substitute's) signature on a paper, form or document that is dated and properly witnessed. For out-of-hospital transfusions, it is desirable to include some acknowledgment of this setting as part of the consent to treatment. For legal purposes, the form provides some evidence of the preceding dialogue but cannot substitute for it. The relationship of the physician and patient and the timing and completeness of the communication that resulted in the treatment at issue are key to helping the judge or jury decide whether the patient actually consented.

Legal Standard for Consent

The standard for determining informed consent has changed. Originally, courts tended to favor the physician, requiring only that informed consent be consistent with what a reasonably prudent professional would expect. However, modern courts have shifted to focus on the patient, rather than the physician. The majority view holds that consent is informed if a reasonable person in the position of the patient would have agreed (*Sard v Hardy*).[7] The minority opinion insists that for consent to be informed, it must be what the reasonable patient him/herself understood when he/she agreed (*Canterbury v Spence*).[8] Clearly, the form alone cannot prove consent was informed.

Shared Responsibilities

The Physician

In the out-of-hospital transfusion setting, the same five duties of a physician apply as in any setting, namely, that the physician must 1) practice at the expected standard of care that training and experience demand, 2) make full disclosure to the patient, 3) protect confidences, 4) seek consultation when indicated and 5) offer continuing treatment.[9] It is incumbent on each transfusing physician to document medical necessity and proper informed consent for treatment when ordering transfusion therapy. Similarly, when the transfusion is to be administered in an out-of-hospital setting, the nuances of the setting itself should be detailed so that it is clear that the physician understands his/her continuing responsibility for care during and after each transfusion event.

If complications of transfusion occur, the treating physician would ordinarily be expected to respond and order additional treatment. If complications resulted from negligence on the part of the supplier or transfuser, physician culpability may be minimized.

Questions of mental competency of the transfusion recipient are also usually the responsibility of the attending physician. Part of the ordering physician's assessment of suitability for out-of-hospital transfusion should include an evaluation of the mental state of the patient and the surroundings in which transfusion would be administered.

The measure of the completeness of a physician's compliance with the medical standard of care is obtained in court via expert testimony of other physicians. Often, the patient's medical record, which contains evidence of written orders for transfusion and of the patient's informed consent, is used to support the physician's claim of nonnegligence. Peer review of out-of-hospital transfusion services, when properly performed, can be helpful in establishing standard of care for such transfusion practices.

The Patient

Patients also have responsibilities in the physician-patient relationship—to disclose fully and to cooperate with an agreed-on treatment plan. Patients who receive out-of-hospital transfusion therapy are often significantly affected by the disease process that necessitates the transfusion. Sometimes, this impairment raises questions of legal competency to consent. The law provides for surrogate decision-making, usually at a local or state level. When the patient is incapacitated such that mentation may be questioned, a legally recognized adult may substitute for the patient in the informed consent process. Careful and thorough documentation of this substitution is prudent.

Patients (and their surrogates) have the right of autonomy and of self-determination (ie, can make decisions about their own bodies) even when those decisions are contrary to medical advice. However, they also are responsible for giving informed consent when they agree with their doctor's advice. Patients requesting out-of-hospital transfusions may so strongly prefer this choice that they minimize or disregard warnings about the enhanced risk. The treating physician should ensure that these additional risks are thoroughly discussed and documented.

The Transfuser and the Supplier

The Transfuser

Transfusing organizations should adhere to existing standards for qualifications and experience of personnel, as well as established standards for procedures and performance (including safety and disposal practices), preferably using the same procedures and practices as the supplying blood center or transfusion service. Beginning with the blood sample collection, complete documentation is prudent.

The location and responsibility for preserving records should be identified in the written agreement between transfuser and supplier.

The Supplier

Blood centers and transfusion services that provide out-of-hospital transfusions have some of the same responsibilities as for in-hospital transfusions—properly receiving the blood sample for crossmatching; maintaining correct records; avoiding errors in the clerical, serologic and technical aspects of crossmatching/compatibility testing; and providing a safe and suitable blood component for each patient. Whether there is additional responsibility for evaluating adequacy of transfusing personnel, policies and procedures and medical oversight of the transfusing facility is unresolved. Because transfusing facilities may be unfamiliar with the legal and regulatory constraints on blood transfusion, courts may rely on the hospital blood bank/transfusion service and/or the blood center for such expertise. However, no litigation has occurred thus far on this question. As would be true for all activities, if the supplier opted to provide additional services to the transfuser, the legal expectation would be that the supplier act reasonably.

Summary

Out-of-hospital transfusion raises important legal questions beyond those of transfusions in the more traditional hospital setting. Because emergency intervention is usually less readily available and the setting may be quite remote, responsibilities differ. When errors occur, response may be inadequate if not defined and understood in advance. The nature and adequacy of informed consent for the procedure may be at issue because of the patient's incapacity, because there was inadequate or incomplete information provided for consent, because someone other than the responsible physician provided the information for consent, and for other reasons. The increased complexity of providing services out-of-hospital creates greater opportunity for negligent behavior, based solely on the number and location of persons involved.

Two legal theories provide the usual basis for action by patients: battery and negligence (medical malpractice). In the out-of-hospital setting, breach of contract may provide an additional basis, particularly among the providers (physicians, transfusers and suppliers). As patients recognize the desirability of out-of-hospital locations for their transfusion therapy, demands for these services will likely increase. Providers should minimize their exposure for liability in these settings by careful prospective attention to preventive measures.

References

1. Rutman RC, Silberstein LE, eds. Out-of-hospital transfusions. Arlington, VA: American Association of Blood Banks, 1986.
2. Widmann FK, ed. Informed consent for blood transfusion. Arlington, VA: American Association of Blood Banks, 1989.
3. Salgo v Leland Stanford Jr. University Board of Trustees et al, 154 CA2d 560, 578, 317 P2d 170,182, 1957.
4. Schloendorff v Society of New York Hospital, 211 NY 125, 105 NE 92, 1914.
5. Cobbs v Grant, 8 Cal3d 229, 104 Cal Rptr 505, 502 P3d 1, 1972.
6. Truman v Thomas, 27 Cal3d 165, 165 Cal Rptr 308, 611 P2d 902, 1980.
7. Sard v Hardy, 281 Md 432, 444, 379 A2d 1014,1020, 1977.
8. Canterbury v Spence, 464 F. 2d 772 (D.C. Circ. 1972).
9. Dornette W. Negligence and liability issues. In: Clark G, ed. Legal issues in transfusion medicine. Arlington, VA: American Association of Blood Banks, 1986:238.

In: Fridey JL, Kasprisin CA and Issitt LA, eds.
Out-of-Hospital Transfusion Therapy
Bethesda, MD: American Association of Blood Banks, 1994

6

Are the Marshals Coming to Dodge City?

Duke O. Kasprisin, MD

THE GROWING ECONOMIC PRESSURE to reduce health-care costs has resulted in an increasing number of medical procedures being performed outside the hospital. Many of these procedures require blood transfusion. Therefore, transfusions are now being given by dialysis centers, outpatient surgical centers, nursing homes, home infusion groups, visiting nurse services, oncology clinics, physicians' offices and numerous other health-care providers.

With the removal of the safety umbrella of hospital-based quality assurance and audit systems, there is a growing concern that transfusion safety may be sacrificed. Numerous questions have arisen as out-of-hospital transfusions become more common. What will be the indications for transfusion in these new settings? Who will audit transfusion practice and who will correct inappropriate usage? Who will train the staff that is administering blood components? Who will investigate transfusion reactions? A plethora of additional concerns could easily be cited.

With the increasing diversity of settings in which blood may be transfused and the variety of health-care professionals who may be involved in the transfusion process, the skill level of the transfusionist will be paramount in maintaining transfusion safety. Will the transfusionists in these new settings understand compatibility and will they recognize serious untoward reactions? If the skill level cannot be guaranteed and significant and possibly life-endangering problems arise, then regulation will quickly follow.

Duke O. Kasprisin, MD, Principal Officer, American Red Cross Blood Services, Vermont/New Hampshire Region, Burlington, Vermont

The risks of grave consequences are very real. For example, transfusions given in the home do not have the advantages of additional skilled help if problems arise; equipment and medications to manage an acute problem will be limited and no laboratory will be readily available to work up problems quickly or to supply a replacement unit of blood if the original unit is discontinued.

The literature concerning the risks of transfusion outside the hospital and the skill level and training of transfusionists is sparse. Therefore, an examination of the problems identified in the hospital setting is pertinent.

This chapter examines some of the potential problems associated with transfusions given outside the hospital setting and the guidelines and regulations that have been created to manage these growing concerns.

Potential Risks

Warnings about the risks of transfusion have appeared in the literature for many years.[1-6] Deaths due to transfusion must be reported to the Food and Drug Administration (FDA) Center for Biologics Evaluation and Research (CBER) by the facility that performed the crossmatch. Reports of these deaths have been reviewed periodically. The most recent evaluation of these reports includes 355 fatalities associated with transfusion between 1976 and 1985.[1] The authors excluded 99 cases that included those not related to transfusion, deaths in donors and deaths due to hepatitis or AIDS where negligence was not a complicating factor.

Of the remaining 256 cases, 51% were directly related to the transfusion of an ABO-incompatible blood component. The vast majority of these were due to errors. Although some of the deaths in which patients received the wrong unit of blood were due to laboratory error, most errors occurred during the initial drawing of a crossmatch specimen or during the administration of blood.

A wide spectrum of errors was identified. In some cases, samples were drawn from the wrong patient because the recipient was not properly identified. In other cases, the patient was correctly identified, but the crossmatch specimen was mislabeled. Another common error was the administration of a properly labeled unit to the wrong patient because of improper identification of the intended patient.

The locations in which these mistakes occurred were diverse, including in surgical suites, intensive care units, emergency rooms and patient wards. When a physician was the sole cause of the error, the most common site was the operating room and anesthesiologists were usually implicated. Nurses were identified as the sole cause in 51 cases, and physicians in 11 others. A common problem identified was the lack of adequate training of the transfusionist in identification procedures.

Within New York, the state regulates blood transfusion services, including "limited transfusion services" (see Appendix 6-1).[7] In December, 1989, the state required that incidents, accidents and errors involving the transfusion of blood components and blood derivatives be reported to the state health department. One hundred and four significant errors were reported by the 285 regulated facilities from January 1, 1990 to October 31, 1991.[8] Fifty-four of these occurrences involved the transfusion of ABO-incompatible red cells. The investigators noted that 58% (61/104) of these mistakes occurred outside the blood bank. Most of these errors were caused by a failure of the transfusionist to identify properly either the recipient or the unit of blood. The process of identifying the unit and the patient is a strictly regulated function in this state.

This study concluded with suggestions to minimize the risk of errors during transfusion. Several of these suggestions would present challenges in the out-of-hospital setting. For example, one suggestion was to require two staff members to identify each unit and recipient. In a clinic or dialysis unit, this practice may cause no problem, but for a transfusion at home would a family member or the patient be an appropriate alternative? The use of two staff members in the home setting may remove the economic advantage of performing this procedure outside the hospital. If regulation of the transfusion process increases, will regulators acknowledge the uniqueness of the out-of-hospital setting and allow alternative methods as New York State has done by allowing the second person checking the identity of the patient to be a family member? Another suggestion from this study was to use commercially available blood bag locking systems. This type of system appears ideal for the home transfusion setting and may offer additional safety when only one staff person is performing the verification of patient identity. However, it should be noted that this is not a foolproof system and there have been anecdotal reports of the occurrence of lock failures.

Based on the number of transfusions given in the State of New York, the authors of this study[8] reported an ABO-incompatible transfusion rate of 1 per 33,000 transfusions. Because ABO-compatible errors are often unrecognized and probably underreported, they estimated that the true transfusion error risk is 1 incident per 12,000 transfusions. This risk level translates into a death rate due to ABO-incompatible transfusions of 1 death per 600,000 transfusions. These figures were comparable to the number of ABO-incompatible transfusion deaths reported to the FDA from 1976-1985—1.43 deaths per million red cell units transfused.

Serious consequences of transfusion errors are relatively uncommon. However, the true number of errors may be quite high. Recently, the College of American Pathologists Laboratory Accreditation Program found that blood transfusion recipients were improperly identified in at least 1.2% of institutions.[9]

Comparing the potential for risk of in-hospital vs out-of-hospital transfusions is difficult. The quality of staff training varies greatly in both settings. Home transfusions may be considered riskier if the staff performs this function infrequently or lacks additional professional help at the scene if a problem arises. On the other hand, transfusion at home involves a 1:1 patient/health professional ratio, which could diminish the distractions of a busy hospital setting and therefore improve safety. However, reviews of reported fatalities prove the potential is present no matter where the transfusion is given.

Training

Regulators are also concerned with the quality, effectiveness and completeness of training for all staff administering blood. In a recent consent decree of permanent injunction with the American National Red Cross,[10] one of the areas of particular concern to the FDA was the adequacy of training. The decree required the monitoring, evaluation and documentation of training for all regulated functions at American Red Cross Blood Service facilities, including adverse reactions from transfusion.

As more and more nonhospital transfusion services are created, how competent can we expect the staff administering the transfusions to be? How knowledgeable are the people who are primarily responsible for transfusing the patient? In general, little time is spent in teaching transfusion therapy in medical or nursing school. It is usually assumed that nurses and physicians will learn about blood components once they are working with patients. If the transfer of knowledge is to be effective, ward nurses and physicians must have a sound knowledge of transfusion therapy themselves and they must be capable of teaching new employees. Because many areas of medicine are taught in this fashion by staff with little or no formal training, it is important to evaluate the knowledge of the persons doing the instruction.

Although errors in transfusion therapy occur too often and a deficit in knowledge among transfusionists concerning blood components has been suspected, concrete data documenting these deficits are scarce. Many studies have been published identifying the sources of error in the laboratory, but few have examined the knowledge deficits of the persons primarily responsible for administering the blood. During the creation of a continuing education program in blood component therapy for physicians and nurses, a university hospital blood bank actually tested the participants to identify what areas should be stressed.[11] The studies revealed several areas of weakness.

When first- and second-year house officers (interns and residents) were tested, it appeared that they learned through experience because residents did somewhat better than the interns. However, numerous inadequacies in overall knowledge were identified in both groups. When nurses were tested, the results were quite similar.[12] The studies revealed that some areas of knowledge were so poor, that if a mistake was made in the laboratory, it was almost assured that it would not be discovered on the wards.

For example, the nurses were given actual hospital blood bag labels to examine and 14% did not recognize an outdated unit. Less than half of the physicians knew what intravenous solutions are compatible with blood administration. Most of the participants had some understanding of red cell compatibility, although many were uncertain about giving Rh-negative red cells to Rh-positive patients. However, very few nurses or physicians were familiar with plasma compatibilities. It appeared that, in general, nurses had greater knowledge concerning blood administration techniques while physicians demonstrated more theoretical knowledge.

Shulman et al[9] studied compliance with their hospital's blood administration practices and found variances committed during 50% of the transfusions. These findings prompted them to create a new compliance program. The transfusion policies and procedures were reviewed at various professional levels, teaching the staff about the problem. The program required a major commitment from the hospital administration as considerable resources were expended to resolve the problem. During a 2-year period, 200 transfusions were audited for compliance with the hospital's procedures. The monitoring created numerous teaching opportunities. When errors occurred, the involved employee was responsible for developing a corrective action plan. If there was an inadequate response by the staff, reminders were generated until there was resolution. Kasprisin[13] has termed this methodology "auditing into compliance," noting that the constant reinforcement led to improvement, reaching 100% compliance over time. However, the study also found a slight decrease in compliance in the audit period, raising questions as to whether it is possible to maintain this level of resource commitment long-term and causing concern that the impact of the program was beginning to deteriorate as staff became complacent to the program. No training method yet identified resolves the problem of proper recipient identification, and variable attention and resource commitment to this problem remain an issue in hospitals.

Blood centers and/or hospital blood banks will probably be linked legally and by regulation to the out-of-hospital facilities they supply. Many of the new types of transfusion sites have actually established much better training and certification of their staff than hospitals, but the skill and documentation are far from uniform. It has been suggested that one way to decrease the risk of transfusion in a home transfusion program is to use only nurses who are trained in the administration of blood. Unfortunately, hospital training of nursing staff in transfusion therapy has been highly variable. The institution of a quality training course, diligent adherence to compliance and consistent auditing programs will be necessary to avoid many of the transfusion problems that have occurred in hospitals. Because out-of-hospital transfusions are provided by facilities that have a more limited scope of therapy than hospitals, quality training and auditing programs can be more effectively established in such settings.

Monitoring the Use of Blood

The question of blood transfusion safety must also include an evaluation of the appropriateness of the transfusion. Monitoring of physicians' use of blood has increased dramatically in the past few years, particularly with the concern over legal liability regarding transfusion-transmitted HIV infection. Although many hospitals had transfusion committees in place, the 1985 requirement by the Joint Commission on Accreditation of Healthcare Organizations (JCAHO) that all transfusions must be audited greatly affected transfusion practice. The American Association of Blood Banks recently published a monograph on quality assurance in transfusion medicine.[14] The publication examines diverse approaches to improving quality, including reviews of retrospective, concurrent and prospective audit strategies. A chapter on quality assurance for out-of-hospital transfusions and designs for auditing transfusions is included. The appropriateness of transfusions in the out-of-hospital setting is another area that regulators may consider necessary to monitor.

Regulation

Few regulations exist concerning transfusion outside the hospital. Many states regulate and/or license nonhospital health-care providers but do not specifically govern blood transfusion. Some home care companies have sought additional certification such as that by JCAHO, and some insurance companies have made certification a requirement for payment. However, in general, few states have chosen to regulate the transfusion process.

Before examining the question of whether increased regulation of out-of-hospital transfusion is desirable and/or likely, it would be valuable to review one of the most comprehensive regulatory policies for out-of-hospital transfusion created by the State of New York.[7] The state defines providers of out-of-hospital transfusion as limited transfusion services (LTSs). LTSs include facilities, home care services agencies, physicians' offices or other entities that transfuse blood and may temporarily store and distribute blood within their own organization but rely on a blood bank which holds a permit in blood services-transfusion to perform laboratory tests required under the law. These regulations attempt to cover most of the potential problems that can arise.

LTSs in New York must have a written agreement for the provision of blood with a facility that has a New York State permit in blood services, specifically, transfusion. This written agreement must specify the responsibilities of each party in ensuring conformity with the law. In addition, the New York Department of Health must approve the agreement. This gives the state control of the entire out-of-hospital industry.

The state also requires each LTS to create a protocol subject to the Department of Health's approval that includes the service's standard operating procedures regarding transfusion and the handling of blood. This protocol must contain information about the transportation and storage of blood, management of adverse reactions, qualifications of personnel, a list of what blood products can be given and administrative techniques.

The state requires the facility that provides the blood to approve the LTS's protocol and requires the transfusion committee of the issuing facility to monitor all transfusions. In addition, the LTS must adhere to the guidelines issued by the Council on Human Blood and Transfusion Services, "Elective Out-of-Hospital Transfusion: Recommended Criteria and Guidelines for Transfusion of Blood Components" (see Appendix 6-2).[15] The state can inspect the LTS sites at its discretion.

The New York regulation demonstrates the extent to which regulatory agencies can control out-of-hospital transfusions. This state has created standards for both the transfusing facility as well as the blood bank providing the blood. These regulations will severely limit the design of out-of-hospital transfusion programs. For example, the LTS must have emergency procedures for specified adverse reactions, requiring a physician to be immediately available for telephone consultation. The LTS must be able to provide adequate facilities for treatment and have arrangements for coverage of adverse reactions 24 hours a day. Because of the risks of blood transfusion, immediate access to a physician is desirable; however, in many LTS programs in other areas of the country have not provided for this. Obviously, the management of these requirements may be different for a home infusion company vs a physician's office.

The facility that provides the blood is required to have a transfusion committee of at least five members which meets at least quarterly to review transfusions of all blood and blood products the facility issues. This requirement includes the review of all intraoperative and postoperative salvage procedures. Blood provided by a hospital blood bank can be monitored by the hospital's transfusion committee. This requirement obligates blood centers that offer this service to have a mechanism in place for review of transfusions as well. Since the review of transfusion usage is good medical practice, blood centers *should* already be performing this role.

To Regulate or Not To Regulate

Thus far, the discussion of problems in the out-of-hospital setting has been predominantly theoretical, and few major difficulties have been documented. Whether problems have occurred in the out-of-hospital setting is not necessarily the basis for creating regulation. Recently, the FDA announced its decision to regulate the tissue transplant industry. The new rules would establish quality assurance standards similar to the ones created to safeguard the blood supply. The FDA commissioner, David A. Kessler, emphasized that in general the tissue supply was safe, but action was being "...taken to head off future problems...."[16] The *existence* of problems is not a prerequisite for regulation, just the *potential* for serious life-threatening risks. Undeniably, out-of-hospital transfusions present such risks.

Concern that the tissue industry is not properly monitored by the federal government has led to proposed legislation. Representative Ron Wyden (D-Oregon), one of the sponsors of this legislation, expressed his concern about tissue transplant by saying, "...What's so ominous about this is there's no structure out there at all...." He likened the tissue market to "...Dodge City before the marshals showed up...."[16]

Although some companies that supply out-of-hospital transfusion have done an excellent job in providing safeguards and extensive training programs, and seek certification such as that from JCAHO, this is not uniform in the industry. In the future, it may become apparent that some LTS programs and home health-care agencies are not observing generally accepted out-of-hospital transfusion practices; this may propel the industry into a regulated environment. It is only a matter of time before the marshals show up in Dodge City.

Acknowledgment

Special thanks are extended to staff at the New York State Department of Health and Laurie Munk at the AABB National Office for assistance in preparing this chapter.

References

1. Sazama K. Reports of 355 transfusion-associated deaths: 1976 through 1985. Transfusion 1990;30:583-90.
2. Myhre BA. Fatalities from blood transfusion. JAMA 1980;244: 1333-5.
3. Honig CL, Bove JR. Transfusion-associated fatalities: Review of Bureau of Biologics Reports 1976-1978. Transfusion 1980;20: 653-61.
4. Schmidt PJ. Transfusion mortality; with special reference to surgical and intensive care facilities. J Fl Med Assoc 1980; 67:151-3.
5. Camp FR, Monaghan WP. Fatal blood transfusion reactions. An analysis. Am J Forensic Med Pathol 1981;2:143-50.

6. Edinger SE. A closer look at fatal transfusion reactions. MLO 1985;April:412-45.
7. Title 10 NYCRR, Part 58, subpart 58-2.
8. Linden JV, Paul B, Dressler KP. A report of 104 transfusion errors in New York State. Transfusion 1992;32:601-6.
9. Shulman IA, Lohr K, Derdiarian AK, Picukaric JM. Monitoring transfusionist practices: A strategy for improving transfusion safety. Transfusion 1994;34:11-15.
10. United States of America v American National Red Cross, No. 93-0949 (D.D.C. May 12, 1993).
11. Kasprisin DO, Kasprisin L. House staff knowledge of blood component therapy: An evaluation. Eval Health Prof 1980; 3:153-8.
12. Kasprisin CA, Kasprisin DO, Marks D, et al. Quality assurance beyond the blood bank. Superv Nurse 1981;12(5):45-8.
13. Kasprisin CA. Auditing into compliance (editorial). Transfusion 1994;34:5-6.
14. Snyder EL, Menitove JE, eds. Home transfusion therapy. Arlington, VA: American Association of Blood Banks, 1986.
15. Council on Human Blood and Transfusion Services. Elective out-of-hospital transfusion: Recommended criteria and guidelines for transfusion of blood components. Albany, NY: New York State Department of Health, 1989.
16. Schwartz J. FDA sets new rules to ensure safety of tissue for transplants. Washington Post Dec. 11, 1993.

Appendix 6-1. New York State Law Regarding Limited Transfusion Services (Title 10 NYCRR, Part 58, Subpart 58-2)[7]

Abbreviated Text Pertaining to Limited Transfusion Services

58-2.1 Definitions- 1. Limited transfusion service means a facility, home care services agency, physician's office, or other entity which transfuses blood and may temporarily store blood and distribute it within its own organization, but relies on a blood bank holding a permit in blood services-transfusion to perform laboratory tests required under section 58-2.17 of this Subpart.

58-2.8 Standard operating procedures.

(a) Current standard operating procedure manuals or other procedural guides specific to the facility shall be available at all times in the immediate work area of personnel engaged in the collection, processing, testing, storage and distribution of blood, blood components or derivatives for autogeneic or allogeneic use, and for therapeutic, prophylactic or diagnostic purposes. There shall be a written protocol for all procedures performed at the facility. Manuals shall contain a protocol for writing, maintaining and periodic review of standard operating procedures by user personnel and management staff. Procedure manuals shall have the following features:
   (1) A standardized format;
   (2) A system of numbering and/or entitling individual procedures;
   (3) A clearly written description of purpose for each procedure;
   (4) A reference section listing appropriate scientific literature;
   (5) Clearly defined areas of personnel responsibility by title;
   (6) Documented approval of procedures and procedural modifications by the director, and annual review by the director or authorized supervisor;
   (7) Instructions for the completion of reports and forms, including examples;
   (8) Effective date and date of review for each procedure; and
   (9) A system of archiving earlier versions of procedures and forms.

(b) The procedure manual shall include a written procedure for documenting errors or accidents in collection, testing, processing, storage or distribution that may affect the safety or purity of any product, or health of the donor or recipient. If the error or accident is not detected prior to issuance of the blood, blood components or derivatives, the error or accident shall be reported immediately to the receiving facility. All such errors and accidents shall also be reported to the department's Wadsworth Center for Laboratories and Research within seven (7) calendar days of discovery.

(c) The procedure manual shall include written policies and protocols regarding the following, for activities performed at the site:
  (1) Use and maintenance of blood warming devices;
  (2) Type of infusion sets and filters for all components;
  (3) Inspection of components prior to issuance;
  (4) Type of personnel who may remove components;
  (5) For collecting facilities, obtaining blood or components from other institutions during emergency situations;
  (6) Prenatal and neonatal testing;
  (7) Evaluation of reported transfusion reactions; and emergency release of uncrossmatched blood.

(d) The policies and procedures specified in the procedure manual shall be followed at all times. If deviations are identified, appropriate corrective action shall be taken and documented.

(e) The blood bank director or the director of transfusion services shall establish and maintain a planned and periodic internal review program for monitoring and evaluating the quality and appropriateness of standard operating procedures in the performance of blood banking activities. Included in the program must be a system for designing and implementing corrective action for any problems identified. Quality assurance deficiencies shall be documented, and evidence shall be available that problems are reported to the appropriate individuals in a timely manner and that corrective action is implemented and subsequently followed-up.

58-2.9 Issuance of blood, blood components and derivatives.

(a) Unless they are needed to meet a medical emergency, blood and blood components shall be transported in a leak-resistant, crush-resistant and puncture resistant container featuring a prominent label which:
  (1) Identifies the contents as "human blood" or "biomedical product";
  (2) Describes the contents, the packing agent, if any, and any special precautions necessary in handling such blood; and

(3) Contains the name, address and twenty-four hour telephone number of the person or entity to be contacted in the event that the container is found leaking, damaged or unattended.

(b) Except in an emergency or except as indicated in section 58-2.3(c) or (d) of this Subpart, blood and blood components shall not be made available for allogeneic transfusion unless a blood sample from the donor reacts negatively to approved tests for syphilis, HBsAg and anti-HBc, and tests for antibodies to hepatitis C virus, HIV-1, HIV-2 and HTLV-I, and has acceptable ALT activity. Untested or incompletely tested blood, including blood from directed donations and cytapheresis collections, shall not be issued if a fully tested blood component is available except in the case of autogenic donations, as specified in section 58 -2.3(a) of this Subpart. Cytapheresis units for which testing has not been completed may be distributed to a hospital by the facility collecting the unit, but such products may not be issued by a transfusion service until testing is complete, except in the case of a life-threatening emergency. The release of cytapheresis products from a donor found to have an unacceptable ALT result or a positive result for anti-HBc, may be permitted upon the authorization of the physician ordering the transfusion and the written authorization of the medical director or other physician designated by the medical director, provided that such authorization documents the indication and justification for such release. Such products shall be labeled with all positive or unacceptable test results. Blood from a donor whose blood sample reacts positively in a test for syphilis and is nonreactive in confirmatory testing shall be appropriately labeled and may be used for plasma fractionation. Blood from a donor whose blood sample reacts positively in tests for antibodies to hepatitis C virus, anti-HBc or HTLV-I and/or has unacceptable ALT activity shall be appropriately labeled and may be used for plasma fractionation. Blood from a donor whose blood sample reacts positively in tests for HBsAg, or antibodies to HIV-1 and/or HIV-2 shall be appropriately labeled and may not be used for allogeneic transfusion or for fractionation. Blood from a donor whose blood sample reacts positively in tests for HBsAg, or antibodies to HIV-1 and/or HIV-2 may not be used for autogeneic transfusion without the written authorization of the patient's physician and, if drawn by another facility, the director of the transfusion service receiving the unit.

(c) Blood components and derivatives shall be issued only if ordered by a licensed physician or other person authorized by law.

Recipients shall receive whole blood of the same ABO group or compatible red blood cells. $Rh_o(D)$-negative recipients shall receive $Rh_o(D)$-negative blood except for reasonable exempting circumstances as determined by the director of transfusion services. $Rh_o(D)$-positive recipients may receive $Rh_o(D)$-positive or $Rh_o(D)$-negative whole blood or red blood cells. In an emergency, appropriately documented in the records, blood may be released for transfusion prior to the completion of compatibility tests. Any transfusion service which issues blood for transfusion at a limited transfusion service shall perform the required tests on its own premises unless the limited transfusion service holds the required permit issued by the department to perform such tests.

(d) Whole blood, red blood cells, plasma or other blood components and derivatives shall be inspected visually immediately prior to issuance. If the color or physical appearance is abnormal or there is indication or suspicion of microbial contamination, the unit or units of whole blood, blood components or derivatives shall not be issued for transfusion.

(e) Blood, blood components or derivatives may not be made available for transfusion beyond the designated expiration date, except that whole blood may be used to prepare plasma within nine days after the designated expiration date, provided that it meets the inspection standards required in subdivision (d) of this section.

(f) An established protocol for processing or pooling of blood components prior to issuance must be in place.

(g) Except in emergency situations, or in case of release to an operating room with a monitored refrigerator, only one unit of red cells at a time may be issued for a particular patient, unless otherwise authorized in writing by the director of transfusion services.

(h) If an unused, unopened unit is returned to the blood bank, the time, date and condition of the unit must be recorded.

(i) A sample of red cells or whole blood from each red cell product issued for transfusion shall be retained for a minimum of seven days after the transfusion for further testing in the event of an adverse reaction.

(j) After issuance, red blood cells may be stored at room temperature for up to one hour or by refrigerating at between one and six degrees Celsius. Red blood cells stored at room temperature for more than 30 minutes may not be returned to the blood bank and later reissued for transfusion unless the temperature of the component is documented not to have risen above six degrees Celsius. If refrigerated, red blood cells shall be stored in a refrigerator designed for the purpose of storing blood, except that a cooler with wet ice may be used for refrigeration, provided that the temperature of the blood is maintained at between one and six degrees Celsius.

(k) Blood or blood components shall not be identified or labeled or preferentially distributed according to the donor's membership in a category based on age, race, color, creed, national origin, sex, marital status or social organization, except for purposes of phenotyping of blood units. The sequence of issuance by a transfusion service of blood donated for designated recipients shall not be based on factors other than medical considerations.

(l) Blood or blood components from a donor who had been determined in the past to be unsuitable for subsequent donation shall not be released for transfusion unless the donor has been approved for reentry into the donor pool by the director of the blood bank.

58-2.10 Required records and confidentiality.

Complete and accurate records of blood, blood components and derivatives released for allogeneic or autogeneic transfusion shall be kept for seven years or six months after the expiration date of the individual product, whichever is later, by the blood bank preparing the product and by the institution using the product. Such records shall be open to inspection by the department and shall include the information specified in sections 58-2.11 and 58-2.12 of this Subpart. For all collected or distributed blood, blood components and derivatives, the donor's name, address, telephone number, social security number and any other information which would directly or indirectly identify the blood donor of any specific unit shall not be disclosed by the blood bank to any person or entity except upon the written consent of the donor or except to the department and other agencies which issue clinical laboratory and/or blood bank permits to the facility whose records are requested.

58-2.12 Records to be kept when blood, blood components or derivatives are issued for allogeneic or autogeneic transfusion.

(a) For blood and blood components, logbook records of the following information, where relevant, shall be kept in the blood bank and made available to the department for inspection:

(1) Source;
(2) Donor identification code;
(3) ABO and Rh groups,
(4) Expiration date;
(5) Results of compatibility tests;
(6) Disposition of the unit including recipient's name if administered;
(7) Signature or initials of the person removing the unit;
(8) Date and time of issue; and
(9) Results of all tests associated with the investigation of all transfusion reactions, with the conclusions reached and the report signed by the director of the blood bank or a qualified physician designated by the director of the blood bank.

(b) For coagulation factor concentrates, logbook records of the following information shall be kept and made available to the department for inspection:
(1) manufacturer;
(2) lot number,
(3) expiration date;
(4) disposition, including recipient's name if administered; and
(5) date of issue.

(c) For all derivatives, records associated with the investigation of all reactions, with the conclusions reached and the report signed by the director of the blood bank or a qualified physician designated by the director of the blood bank, shall be kept and made available to the department for inspection.

(d) These recordkeeping requirements shall also apply to blood issued to limited transfusion services.

58-2.16 Required standards for transfusions.

(a) Transfusion services. Every institution which performs transfusions or supplies blood to limited transfusion services shall designate a physician who is a member of the staff as director of transfusion services. Such physician must be licensed and currently registered in New York State. The director of the blood bank, if a physician, may be so designated. The premises, equipment, procedure manuals, records, and all blood, blood components and derivatives shall be available for inspection by the department.
(1) It shall be the responsibility of the chief executive officer or other person in charge of each institution and of the director of transfusion services to determine that:

(i) The rules and regulations of the Council on Human Blood and Transfusion Services and the Administrative Rules and Regulations of the department and related requirements are complied with;

(ii) Attending and other staff members and nurses are properly instructed regarding all required procedures;

(iii) Records required by the aforesaid rules and regulations are maintained;

(iv) Serious unexpected reactions and incidents involving transfusions are reported to the department's Wadsworth Center for Laboratories and Research, on a form approved by the department with sufficient detail to facilitate evaluation and investigation within seven (7) calendar days of the reaction or incident or its discovery; and

(v) A written policy exists regarding use of blood components negative for cytomegalovirus antibody, irradiated components, leukoreduced components and other specialty components. Such a policy shall include recommended indications for component use and a protocol for component processing and issuance. There shall also be a written policy on recommended indications for transfusion of whole blood, fresh frozen plasma and platelets.

(2) The institution shall report annually to the department the name(s) of the physician(s) in charge of the transfusion service.

(3) If blood is issued to a limited transfusion service, the director of transfusion services of the issuing facility and the director of the limited transfusion service performing the transfusion shall ensure compliance with all requirements of this Part.

(b) Each facility which transfuses blood or supplies blood to limited transfusion services shall have a transfusion committee which meets at least quarterly or more frequently as required by the department. The committee shall:

(1) Be composed of at least five members, a majority of whom are present at each meeting;

(2) Include members with expertise in transfusion medicine and qualified to review the appropriateness and technical aspects of a transfusion, such as, but not limited to, the director of transfusion services, blood bank supervisor or pathologist; and

(3) Review transfusions of all blood and blood products issued by the facility for all sites at which transfusions are performed, including all intraoperative and postoperative salvage procedures.

(c) Each institution, through its transfusion committee, shall establish guidelines for reservation (compatibility or crossmatching) of blood for each elective surgical procedure which has been performed there more than five times in the preceding calendar year and shall set the maximum number of hours that cross matched blood will be held on reserve.

(d) Whole blood, red blood cells, plasma, or other components and derivatives shall be prepared and administered by methods generally accepted by the FDA or American Association of Blood Banks and/or by other methods approved by the department as in conformance with generally accepted laboratory principles. For blood and blood components, the person performing the transfusion must be a physician, registered nurse, physician's assistant or nurse practitioner. A filter meeting FDA requirements shall be incorporated into the intravenous administration set to be used for blood or blood component transfusions.

(e) No medications except physiologic saline for intravenous use shall be added to or mixed with blood for transfusion.

(f) Immediately prior to the administration of a blood product, the person administering the blood product and one additional person other than the recipient, shall, at the patient site, positively identify the recipient and the blood product to be transfused or infused, unless another procedure to ensure accurate identification is used in which case a single identification is sufficient. Each identification procedure shall be documented in writing.

(g) The person administering the transfusion and another competent adult, other than the recipient, shall be immediately available at all times during a transfusion. Transfusion staff shall be available for 30 minutes afterwards, except for transfusions of patients enrolled in a chronic transfusion program who have no history of adverse reactions.

(h) Every facility or limited transfusion service performing transfusions shall provide 24-hour-a-day post-transfusion patient coverage by telephone as necessary.

(i) Each institution, through its transfusion committee, shall develop and implement procedures to encourage the use of autogeneic blood whenever medically indicated. These procedures shall include a mechanism for informing staff physicians of the risks and benefits of autogeneic blood and the options for autogeneic blood transfusion available at the institution. These procedures shall also include a mechanism to encourage physicians to inform their patients of such options whenever medically indicated.

58-2.17 Laboratory tests to be performed prior to allogeneic or autogeneic transfusion.

(a) Tests shall be performed to determine the ABO and Rho (D) groups of each recipient and each unit to be transfused in accordance with procedures approved by the department pursuant to this Subpart. ABO grouping tests shall include both forward and reverse grouping except in the case of a hospital transfusion services verifying a blood group determination performed elsewhere, in which case forward grouping alone may be performed. The transfusion service performing a crossmatch must confirm the ABO group of all units of whole blood and red cell components, as well as the Rh group of all such units labeled as Rh-negative, using a sample obtained from an attached segment. Any discrepancies shall be reported in writing to the collecting facility and resolved prior to issuance of the blood for transfusion purposes.

(b) All recipient blood shall be tested for unexpected alloantibodies using reagent red blood cells that meet FDA standards, are intended for this purpose and are not pooled. Methods of testing for unexpected alloantibodies shall demonstrate sensitizing and hemolytic antibodies.

(c) Except in cases necessitating emergency release of group-compatible blood or except in the case of transfusion of a volume of blood or blood components exceeding the recipient's expected normal blood volume in a 24-hour period, compatibility between recipient and donor blood shall be determined. If a clinically significant antibody has been detected, or if there is a history of presence of such an antibody, the compatibility test must include an antiglobulin phase crossmatch. If no clinically significant antibody has been detected, and there is no known history of presence of such an antibody, the procedure to be used may be determined by the director of transfusion services, but must, at minimum, consist of an immediate spin test or verification of the blood group of the recipient, and of the blood or blood component to be transfused.

(d) In the case of patients requiring repeated blood transfusions or those pregnant or transfused within the previous three months, fresh blood specimens shall be drawn for compatibility testing and antibody screening at intervals of not more than 72 hours prior to a transfusion, except for neonates, to whom no time limits apply.

(e) Each reagent, including test red blood cells, test sera and anti-human globulin, shall be stored in labeled containers under conditions appropriate for such reagent and shall be removed from use after its date of expiration. The reactivity, specificity and potency of each reagent shall be determined whenever a new lot is employed.

(f) All tests, including but not limited to ABO and Rho (D) grouping, antibody detection and identification and compatibility testing, shall employ methods, techniques or procedures which have been recommended for the particular reagent in use by the FDA or the American Association of Blood Banks and been demonstrated to be effective in a manner acceptable to the department as in conformance with generally accepted laboratory principles. All blood grouping sera, reagents, devices, methods and procedures shall conform to the recommended requirements of the FDA.

(g) Records shall be maintained of all tests, controls, reagents and current procedures, in a manner acceptable to the department. Negative controls on each day of use are not required for anti-human globulin and antibody screening cells, provided manufacturers' instructions are followed. New lots of reagents must be thoroughly evaluated, but each shipment of antibody identification cell panels need not be tested with a known antibody. All procedures are to be determined by the blood bank director and must be documented in the standard operating procedure manual. If no negative reactions are observed on a given test run, an investigation must be performed and controls run. Such records shall be accessible to laboratory personnel engaged in immunohematology testing and to the department.

(h) The procedure to be used for compatibility testing is to be determined by the blood bank director, but must, at a minimum, consist of an immediate spin, or verification of the blood group of the recipient and of the blood or blood component to be transfused. Antiglobulin phase compatibility testing is required if a clinically significant antibody is detected during the antibody screen or if there is a history of presence of such an antibody. Laboratory procedure manuals must be revised to reflect any changes in such procedures.

(i) Centrifuges used for testing of red blood cell agglutination shall be calibrated quarterly, and the optimal centrifugation conditions shall be indicated. A microscope shall be located in the work area designated for immunohematology testing. Microscopic examination shall be performed in red blood cell agglutination tests whenever indicated by the procedure in use. There must be documentation that maintenance is performed at least annually to ensure proper operation.

(j) A pretransfusion sample of recipient blood, including serum or plasma, shall be retained for seven days after each transfusion for further testing in the event of an adverse reaction.

58-2.18 Records to be kept when blood or blood component transfusions are performed. The following information shall be included on the recipient's chart or in records maintained in the blood bank:

(a) Donor's identification code;
(b) Donor's ABO and Rh groups;
(c) Date of the transfusion and quantity of material transfused;
(d) Time of starting and time of completing the transfusion;
(e) Description of the blood product;
(f) Description of any adverse reaction and the results of investigations related to this reaction; and
(g) Name(s) of the person(s) who performed the transfusion and who attended the recipient during the transfusion.
(h) In the case of emergency issuance of uncrossmatched blood, the signature of the physician authorizing such emergency release.

58-2. 19 Records to be kept when plasma derivatives are infused. The following information shall be included on the recipient's chart or in records maintained in the blood bank or pharmacy:

(a) Date of infusion and quantity of material infused;
(b) Time of starting and time of completing the infusion;
(c) Description of the plasma derivative, including the name of the fractionating facility or manufacturer, the lot number or other identification, and the expiration date;
(d) Description of any adverse reaction and the results of investigations related to this reaction; and
(e) Names(s) of the person(s) who performed the infusion and who attended the recipient during the infusion.

58-2. 21 Limited transfusion services.

(a) Limited transfusion services shall comply with the provisions in this Part governing transfusions in general.

(b) Limited transfusion services shall have a written agreement with an issuing facility holding a permit in blood services-transfusion. The agreement shall specify the division of responsibilities for assuring conformity with the provisions of this Part. The agreement shall be subject to the prior approval of the department. An inspection may be conducted prior to departmental approval. The agreement must include:

(1) The written approval of the issuing facility's director of transfusion services and the director of the limited transfusion service;

(2) The procedures for transport and storage of blood and means to assure compliance with such procedures:

(3) A description of the transfusion committee of the issuing facility, its responsibilities and composition;

(4) Procedures for training of personnel at the limited transfusion service;

(5) Requirements for handling adverse reactions, including training of personnel, availability of a physician, 24-hour coverage, and reporting and investigation of such reactions;

(6) Procedures for administration of transfusions including staffing requirements; and

(7) Recordkeeping procedures as required in sections 58-2.12, 582.18 and 58-2.19 of this Subpart, clearly describing responsibility for maintenance of records and their location.

(c) Transfusions may be performed outside of hospitals only if the patient is cooperative, able to respond to verbal commands and able to give informed consent. Such patients must have a history of previous uncomplicated transfusion, including absence of hemolytic or anaphylactic reactions. Transfusions may be performed in a patient's home only if physical limitations or hardships exist which would impede transportation to or transfusion in a hospital or ambulatory setting.

(d) A qualified licensed physician must supervise personnel administering transfusions by limited transfusion services and must be responsible for ensuring that such personnel have adequate training and experience.

(e) A licensed physician must be immediately available for personal or telephone consultation during the transfusion and for 30 minutes afterward.

(f) Any site at which a transfusion is performed by a limited transfusion service must have available an accessible working telephone to allow communication with the physician in case of an adverse reaction. All medications, equipment and supplies necessary for the management of adverse reactions must be immediately available on the premises. Infectious waste disposal must be undertaken using containers and procedures found acceptable by the department pursuant to Part 70 of this title.

(g) Referral of a patient for out-of-hospital transfusion therapy must be approved by the director of the limited transfusion service or his/her designee. Each such transfusion must be ordered by a licensed physician, and a copy of the order must be provided to both the limited transfusion service and the facility issuing the blood.

58-2.24 Disposal of untransfused and expired blood units. Units deemed unsuitable for transfusion, those not transfused for any reason, and those designated for disposal for any reasons, shall be disposed of by an appropriate method in accordance with all applicable regulations and requirements. All expired blood components shall be transferred to a separate storage location within 24 hours of expiration. All such components shall be destroyed, discarded, or removed for nontransfusion purposes within 72 hours of expiration, or returned to the collection facility within one week of expiration.

Section 58-2.1 Definitions.

(a) Blood bank means a facility for the collection, processing, storage or distribution of human blood, human blood components or blood derivatives, or the performance of reinfusion procedures. A blood bank shall employ a qualified director for administrative purposes and, if blood collection is performed, a qualified medical director.

(b) Blood donation center means a facility, fixed or mobile, that is operated by a blood bank and used for the collection of blood, plasma or cytapheresis products, or separation of whole blood into components.

(c) Donor or blood donor means a person who provides his/her blood or plasma for transfusion of whole blood, blood components or derivatives.

(d) Blood components means those preparations separated from a single donation of whole blood, or a cytapheresis or plasmapheresis product, intended for use as final products for transfusion, including but not limited to plasma, fresh frozen plasma, red blood cells, washed red blood cells, leukocyte-reduced red blood cells, platelets and cryoprecipitate.
(e) Derivatives means those preparations separated from plasma derived from multiple donors, including but not limited to albumin, immune globulin, plasma protein fraction and clotting factor concentrates.
(f) Blood products means whole blood, blood components or derivatives.
(g) Plasmapheresis means the withdrawal of blood to obtain plasma with subsequent or simultaneous reinfusion into the donor of his/her own red blood cells.
(h) Serial plasmapheresis program means a program of individual donor donations on a regular basis by plasmapheresis yielding three liters or more of plasma per consecutive four-week period.
(i) Cytapheresis means the separation and collection of blood cells by hemapheresis for the purpose of obtaining a transfusable blood component.
(j) Intraoperative blood salvage means salvage of blood from a surgical field and processing of salvaged blood for direct reinfusion, storage or infusion into a cardiac bypass pump. Intraoperative blood salvage does not include performance of perioperative hemodilution procedures. Postoperative blood salvage means salvage of blood from a wound following surgery, and processing of salvaged blood for direct reinfusion or storage.
(k) FDA means the Food and Drug Administration of the United States Department of Health and Human Services.
(l) Limited transfusion service means a facility, home care services agency, physician's office, or other entity which transfuses blood and may temporarily store blood and distribute it within its own organization, but relies on a blood bank holding a permit in blood services-transfusion to perform laboratory tests required under section 58-2.17 of this Subpart.
(m) Holding facility means a facility at which blood is temporarily stored but which does not offer any other blood banking services.
(n) Transfusion service means a service which issues blood or blood components for administration into a person, but does not include a limited transfusion service.
(o) Institution means a hospital or other facility operating a transfusion service under a permit issued by the department or by the New York City Department of Health.

(p) Allogeneic collection means the removal and storage of blood or blood components from a donor for transfusion into another person, and includes blood donated for directed donation to another person, or donated for autogeneic use and subsequently crossed-over for use by others. Allogeneic collection was formerly termed homologous collection.
(q) Autogeneic collection means the removal and storage of blood or blood components from a donor for subsequent reinfusion into that same person, and includes preoperative hemodilution procedures if at any time the blood leaves the operating room in which surgery is performed. Autogeneic collection was formerly termed autologous collection.
(r) Directed donation means an allogeneic collection in which blood from a particular donor is designated for use by a specified recipient.
(s) Medical director means a qualified physician licensed to practice medicine and currently registered under the laws of the State of New York or in the state of practice and who is employed by a blood bank and is responsible for donor selection and safety.
(t) Department means the New York State Department of Health.
(u) Reinfusion procedure means the withdrawal of a small amount of blood or a component thereof from a patient, its processing by addition of substances or by culturing, and reinfusion of the product so obtained, in whole or in part, into the same patient for diagnostic or therapeutic purposes. Reinfusion procedures shall include, but not be limited to, radioisotopic tagging, and genetic and immunologic manipulation, but shall not include the processing of whole blood units into components for autogeneic reinfusion, such as platelet concentrates, packed red blood cells and plasma.

Appendix 6-2. Elective Out-of-Hospital Transfusion: Recommended Criteria and Guidelines for Transfusion of Blood Components[15]

NOTE: This is not applicable to plasma derivatives.

I. Patient Criteria

A. The patient must be cooperative, able to respond to verbal commands and able to give informed consent.
B. The patients should have a history of previous uncomplicated transfusion, including an absence of hemolytic or severe allergic reactions.
C. Stable cardiorespiratory status. Patients with unstable angina or congestive heart failure are not suitable candidates for out-of-hospital transfusion.
D. The patient must meet the transfusion therapy guidelines of the issuing facility for chronic anemia. Appropriate diagnoses include anemias of primary or secondary bone marrow failure. Patients suffering acute blood loss should not be transfused at home.
E. For home transfusion, physical limitations or hardship that would make transportation to or transfusion in a hospital or ambulatory setting difficult.

II. Staffing

A. In addition to physicians, qualified medical personnel such as registered nurses and registered physician's assistants shall start, administer and monitor the transfusions. At least two competent adults, other than the recipient, shall be present at all times during the transfusions, and for 30 minutes afterwards, one of whom is either a physician or suitably trained registered nurse or registered physician's assistant. The supervisory physician must certify that the personnel administering the transfusion have adequate training and experience.
B. If a physician is not present on site during the transfusion, the personnel administering the transfusion must meet the follow-

ing requirements for training and experience. Training and experience shall be suitably documented and include:

1. Experience with acute patient care in a hospital setting
2. Demonstrated skills in venipuncture and IV therapy
3. Completion of an in-service educational program covering all aspects of blood transfusion therapy, preferably including CPR training.

C. If not present on site, a physician must be immediately available by telephone during the transfusion and for 30 minutes afterwards. In an office setting, it is preferable that a physician be present. If this is not possible, personnel must meet the requirements specified in II.B. In all cases, staff must also be available for 24-hour follow-up coverage.

III. Equipment/Supplies

A. All medications, equipment and supplies necessary for the management of adverse reactions must be immediately available.
B. Approved containers and procedures for infectious waste disposal must be used.
C. There must be an accessible working telephone at the location of the transfusion to permit ready communication with the supervising physician.

IV. Transfusion Procedures

The Council on Human Blood and Transfusion Services endorses the transfusion, blood sample collection, blood component administration and transfusion reaction protocols contained in the American Association of Blood Banks' brochure "Out-of-Hospital Transfusions" (publication #BRP 1060) and recommends that these protocols be followed.

Revised 7/3/89

Index

Italicized page numbers indicate tables or figures